Patient to Patient:

Managing Interstitial Cystitis
& Overlapping Conditions

Patient to Patient:

Managing Interstitial Cystitis & Overlapping Conditions

Gaye Grissom Sandler
Andrew B. Sandler, Ph.D.

The material contained in this publication is neither intended nor implied to be given as medical advice. This publication is not intended to serve as a substitute for medical care or consultation with your physician. The information contained herein has been gathered from multiple sources with the intention of sharing this wide-range of information. Great effort has been made to give proper credit to all sources. If you have additional questions, please consult your physician or medical practitioner.

Various trademarked products and names are printed in this book. They are used in an editorial fashion with no intention of infringement of the trademark.

First edition 3000 copies

Library of Congress Catalog Card Number: 00-93537

ISBN: 0-9705590-0-3

Illustrations: Dion Roberts
Graphic Design: Sally Richards
Cover Design and Prepress: Martin/Greater Communications,
                                     New Orleans

Published By:
Bon Ange LLC
5721 Magazine St.
P.M.B. 124
New Orleans, LA 70115

Printed in the United States by
Morris Publishing
3212 E. Hwy 30
Kearney, NE 68847
1-800-650-7888

INTRODUCTION

I am not a doctor and I do not pretend to practice medicine. What I am is an IC patient and I do live the consequences of IC every day of my life. I have lived with this chronic disease for many years and I have learned.

This book is a compilation of my experiences, both good and bad; transcripts, books, and newsletters pulled here through years of research; historic and newly released studies, my husband's perspective and feelings about this disease; shared group experiences, as well as the stories other IC patients across the country have disclosed to me. What I have found, and many of my peers agree, that IC is more than a chronic disease, it is a learning process.

When I was first diagnosed with IC I thought I would get a prescription for some medicine and get on with my life. I was not aware that I was just beginning to deal with a tenacious and unpredictable disease.

A few months after my initial diagnosis, I learned that IC was mostly a woman's disease and that most treatments were in the early stages of research and development. It quickly became apparent that my doctor and I would have to work together to deal with the challenges of this newly recognized disease.

What I have discovered and repeatedly stress in this book, is that finding the right doctor, treatment and/or medication is an individual process and one that may take a long time. On the other hand, the pain and other symptoms of IC often demand immediate attention. This situation leaves IC patients feeling alone, confused and in pain far too long. However, through my personal struggle and review of ongoing research, I have come to understand that IC patients can learn how to manage their lives with more awareness and a sense of control if given information and resources.

Among the resources an IC patient may need are multiple medical practitioners. Although a diagnosis of IC does not necessarily indicate the presence of another disease, many IC patients end up seeking relief and treatment from an array of specialists due to the variety of problems that can accompany IC. Most patients understand that doctors and other healthcare professionals are also frustrated with IC, and soon learn that there is little known research documenting the multiple symptoms of IC. A collaborative approach is required.

Collaborating and sharing is the heart of *Patient to Patient: Managing Interstitial Cystitis and Overlapping Conditions* with the goal of speeding and supporting the learning curve of others who are either newly diagnosed with IC or have been battling it for years. In order to accommodate the individual and unique needs of the IC patient, this book covers a broad spectrum of accompanying symptoms, disorders, self-help strategies, and medical interventions. The focus of *Patient to Patient: Managing Interstitial Cystitis and Overlapping Conditions* is on the many aspects of the patient's life, suggesting a multidisciplinary approach to help improve the quality of life for the individual IC patient, family and friends.

ACKNOWLEDGMENTS

We thank the following IC patients for their contribution, support and encouragement: Molly Hanna Glidden, Sally Berman, Candace Pierce Lavin, Mary Ellen Thompson, Jill Osborne and Bev Laumann.

We are grateful to: our editor, Sara Caskey Smith; movement pioneer, Judith Aston; Merrilee Kullman, P.T., Sylvi Beaumont, D.C., Russell Wilson, Ph.D., Francis Santorelli, Ellen Hermanos, Patte Ryan, Sally Richards, Betty Anglin, Liz Smith, Melissa O'Brien, Margaret Einhorn, Stefania Tosti, Rob Heifner, Charlie and Mary Foxwell, Annie Breaux, Stephanie Rousseau and Kolleen Herndon.

We also wish to express our gratitude to our families and to the medical doctors who have been helpful, particularly Kathleen Walsh and Beverly Yount.

CONTENTS

Contents

Chapter 1
WHAT IS INTERSTITIAL CYSTITIS?

What is Interstitial Cystitis?

Interstitial cystitis (IC) is a chronic, painful inflammatory disease that affects the bladder wall. IC is not a common urinary tract infection. IC is not caused by stress. It is not a psychosomatic disorder. IC can be a debilitating disease and is a recognized disability under the Americans with Disabilities Act (ADA).*

The term interstitial cystitis refers to inflammation within the bladder wall, the space between the bladder lining and the bladder muscle which is called the interstitium.

* *"The ruling of the Sixth Circuit Court that IC is clearly a disability under the ADA has significant implications for IC patients who encounter job discrimination because of their disease"* (*ICA Update*, Fall 1996).

What are the Symptoms of IC?

- Urgency and urinary frequency-15 to 70 times a day, including nocturia (frequency during the night)
- Decreased urine flow
- Pain and burning during and/or after voiding
- Sense of relief during and/or after voiding
- Pain in the bladder, in the urethra, and in and around the pelvic area and the supporting muscles of the pelvic floor (IC pain may occur in women in the vagina, rectum, and perineum - the area between the anus and vagina. Men may feel

1

IC pain in the penis, rectum, scrotum, and perineum - the area between the anus and scrotum. Pain may radiate into the joints and muscles of the low back and sacral area, hips and legs, and affect other areas of the body.)

- IC symptoms may be misdiagnosed as urethritis in women.
- IC symptoms may be misdiagnosed as chronic non-bacterial prostatitis in men
- Patients may mistake IC symptoms for an acute urinary infection

Some patients have a rapid onset of IC symptoms while others may have mild symptoms for a long period of time. These patients may be misdiagnosed until symptoms become chronic. IC symptoms vary patient to patient and can be mild, moderate or severe. The pain of IC has been compared to an abscessed tooth, a migraine, ground glass, paper cuts, a lit match, a twisting knife, acid in the bladder, and the pain of late stage bladder cancer. According to a standard medical tool, the McGill Pain Inventory, the pain of interstitial cystitis was found to be more severe than the pain of advanced (bladder) cancer Whatever the symptoms, the pain of IC can have similarly debili tating effects.

What Causes IC?

No one knows the cause of IC. Some researchers believe that IC is a symptom complex which may have a variety of causes Currently under research are several theories for the cause of inflammation of the bladder wall including:

- Defect in the bladder lining (glycosaminoglycan or GAG layer) which allows toxins in the urine to come into contact with the bladder wall causing inflammation of the tissue and exposed nerves (Often the presence of even a small amount of urine causes the bladder to contract.) *

- Malfunction of the immune system
- Toxins remaining in the system after an illness
- Hormonal imbalance
- Malfunction in the central nervous system which results in a smooth muscle dysfunction (The bladder and urethra are in part smooth muscle.)
- Pathogenic role of mast cells in the bladder (Activation of mast cells plays a part in allergic reactions.)
- Fibromyalgia (FMS) of the bladder
- Bacterial presence between the bladder lining and bladder muscles, within the bladder wall (This bacterial DNA differs from the microorganisms found in regular bladder infections.)
- Irritated nerve endings from previous bacterial infections (Some research has shown that a majority of IC patients have suffered with previous bladder infections.)
- Repeated antibiotic use was once thought to damage the bladder wall
- Other suggested causes include viral, vascular, structural, and exposure to certain unknown environmental substances

* A *1999 ICA Physician Perspective noted that Dr. Susan Keay of the University of Maryland has isolated a peptide-antiproliferative factor (APF) in the urine of many IC patients. APF seems to inhibit the normal growth of bladder epithelial cells which protect the bladder from injury and inflammation (such as a bladder infection). Keay also suggests that exposure to irritating urine contents could trigger a low-level autoimmune response.*

Who is Affected?

An estimated 750,000 Americans have IC. Ninety percent are women. The usual onset of the disease is 30 to 40 years of age, with the average age of the IC patient at 40. However, IC is on the rise in younger people and can affect children.

How is IC Treated?

- Oral medications to create a protective lining on the bladder wall
- Catheterization of the bladder (with a pediatric catheter) and instillation of medications that soothe inflammation and repair the bladder lining or act as a temporary replacement for the bladder lining
- Dietary restrictions - avoiding acidic and spicy foods, as well as other foods containing certain amino acids or amines (The IC patient's bladder has surface damage and leaks and/or can become swollen and irritated after eating foods in these categories.)
- Antidepressants to block pain and aid sleep
- Antispasmodics to calm spasms
- Analgesics to stop burning
- Antihistamines to suppress mast cell activity
- Anti-inflammatory medications to reduce inflammation
- Anti-anxiety medications to calm the pain
- Alpha blockers to block pain and relax smooth muscle
- Estrogen replacement therapy
- Medication to alkalize the urine
- Electric stimulation and biofeedback
- Calcium channel antagonist to inhibit vascular smooth muscle contraction (This treatment is being tested to help bladder capacity.)
- Narcotic antagonist to block mast cell degranulation
- Nerve block to prevent painful nerve impulses
- Denervation to decrease bladder sensation
- Bladder training to increase the intervals between urination

- Alternative treatments used alone or in conjunction with medical treatments
- Surgery - which is considered a last resort

What Causes IC Symptoms to Flare?

Each IC patient is unique. What bothers one patient does not bother another, but there are common irritants. Flare-ups are most frequently associated with:

- Menstrual cycle, perimenopause and menopause
- Diet
- Sexual intercourse
- Allergies and chemical sensitivities to certain medications and chemical fumes
- Stress
- Exercise
- Travel, including riding in a car

Is IC Genetic?

There appears to be a genetic association in some instances and research is ongoing to determine if there is a recessive gene. The presence of an antiproliferative factor in the urine of IC patients may result from a genetic factor.

Is IC Contagious?

There is no evidence that IC is contagious.

HOW CAN WE FIND OUT MORE ABOUT IC?

Organizations:

Interstitial Cystitis Network
(707) 538-9442
www.ic-network.com

Interstitial Cystitis Association (ICA)
51 Monroe Street
Suite 1402
Rockville, Maryland 20850
(301) 610-5300
1-800-ICA-1626
www.ichelp.org

National Bladder Foundation
P.O. Box 1095
Ridgefield, CT 06877
(203) 431-0005
www.bladder.org

National Kidney And Urologic Diseases
Information Clearinghouse
(IC fact sheets are available at no charge.)
NIDDK/ OCPL
31 Center Drive
Room 9A04
Bethesda, MD 20892-3580
(301) 496-3583
www.niddk.nih.gov/index.html

American Foundation for Urologic Disease
The Bladder Health Council
1128 North Charles Street
Baltimore, MD 21201
(410) 468-1800 or 1-800-242-2383

Canada
Canadian Interstitial Cystitis Society (CICS)
Sociètè Canadienne de la cystite interstitielle
Attn: Sandy McNicol - President
P.O. Box 28625
4050 E. Hastings St.
Burnaby, BC V5C 2H0
Canada
Phone: 250.758.3207
Fax: 250.758.4894
E-mail: smcnicol@pacificcoast.net

Germany
ICA Deutschland e.V.
Attn: Barbara Muendner-Hensen—Chair
Untere Burg 21
D-53881 Euskirchen
Germany
Phone: +49.2251.76729
Fax: +49.2251.76729
Internet: www.ica-ev.de

United Kingdom
Interstitial Cystitis Support Group (ICSG)
Attn: Anthony Walker—National Coordinator
76 High Street
Stony Stratford
Buckinghamshire
MK11 1AH
United Kingdom
Phone: +44.1908.569169
Fax: +44.1908.569169
E-mail: info@interstitialcystitis.co.uk
Internet: www.interstitialcystitis.co.uk

The Netherlands
Interstitial Cystitis Patient's Association of the Netherlands (ICPA-NL)
Attn: Jane Meijlink—Chair
B.L.F. de Montignylan 73
3055 NA Rotterdam
The Netherlands
Phone: +31.10.4613330
Fax: +31.10.2857158
E-mail: jane.meijlink@gironet.nl

New Zealand
New Zealand IC Support Group
Attn: Dot Milne, R.N.
Urology Support Services
P.O. Box 33-264
Christchurch
New Zealand
Phone: +64.3.3294005

Books:

The Interstitial Cystitis Survival Guide
Robert Moldwin, M.D. (2000)
Available through the IC Network and the ICA
New Harbinger Publications, Inc.

Overcoming Bladder Disorders
Rebecca Chalker and Kristine Whitmore, M.D. (1990)
Harper Perennial. Available through Barnesandnoble.com
1-800-242-7737

Interstitial Cystitis
Grannum Sant, M.D. (1997)
Lippincott-Raven Publishers, Philadelphia, PA
To order call 1-800-777-2295
Also available through the ICA and Barnesandnoble.com

The ICN Patient Handbook and Workbook
J. Osborne, D. Manhattan
Interstitial Cystitis Network Publishers
To order call (707) 538-9442
www.ic-network.com
Printed and bound copies available
No fee via the IC Network

Interstitial Cystitis
Phillip Hanno, M.D. and David R. Staskin, M.D.(1990)
Springer, Verlag
Available through the ICA

Evaluating and Managing Interstitial Cystitis
Lowell Parsons, M.D.
University Research Association, RX., Inc.,
560 Sylvan Avenue
Englewood Cliffs, NJ O7632
To order call (201) 816-0110 (no fee)

Other books on IC will be mentioned in the chapters to follow.

What is the History of IC?

IC has been known to medicine for a long time. At the turn of the century IC was named Hunner's disease after a doctor who discovered ulcers on the bladder wall of a patient. However, the male-oriented field of urology largely considered IC a rare disorder of post-menopausal women, as well as a malady caused by hysteria. Hysteria was at that time a diagnosis often used for unexplained symptoms and an array of misunderstood illnesses, predominantly affecting women and thought to be caused by repressed emotions. Even later, symptoms of IC were attributed to emotional problems when urine tests came back negative for infection and there were no signs of Hunner's ulcers.

In the 1970's Hunner's ulcers were recognized as rare in patients and not necessary for a diagnosis of IC. By the mid-80's, workshops which were held by the *National Institute for Diabetes, Digestive and Kidney Diseases (NIDDK)* produced the guidelines for selecting people for studies of the treatment for IC. Diagnostic guidelines for IC were established thanks to prominent urologists.

Unfortunately, up until this time, medical schools and textbooks continued to teach and attribute the symptoms of IC to the old theories. The trickle down effect from the theory of hysteria has created biased opinions of IC in both traditional and alternative medicine. It is not unusual for IC patients to visit doctor after doctor before finding a correct diagnosis and effective treatment. Because this situation takes a toll on many patients, it's important for IC patients to find the right doctor who understands the dynamics of IC.

What is the Research on IC?

Research, a renewed interest in IC and education for both physicians and patients have been available since 1987 thanks to the efforts of non-profit organizations including the *Interstitial Cystitis Association (ICA)* and the *American Foundation for Urologic Disease's Bladder Health Council.*

The ICA has testified before the U.S. Senate and the House Health Appropriations Subcommittees to request federal funding for research, education for doctors and money to research diagnostic tools and treatments. Due in part to the ICA's effort, Congress and the *National Institutes of Health (NIH)* directed the NIDDK to research IC. Associations such as the ICA and the *National Bladder Foundation (NBF)* are working cooperatively to achieve higher levels of research funding at the NIH.

There are many good doctors studying IC and an excellent group of doctors on the ICA Medical Advisory Board. As a result, patients have a better chance for a faster diagnosis and treatment than ever before. Even so, research is not easy and more is needed. Research studies often require participants to try a new drug, placebo, different foods, or undergo biopsy. These procedures are impossible for many patients with painful bladder symptoms. Patients with mild IC may be more likely to participate in studies, but may not contribute an accurate picture of the disease for patients with more severe symptoms. Many IC patients cannot consider being part of a study.

How is IC Diagnosed?

To obtain a correct diagnosis of IC it is best to find a urologist who is familiar with IC. The doctor will take a history of symptoms and perform comprehensive urological, neurological and urogynecological evaluations to rule out infections and other possible causes. When all other causes are ruled out, the doctor will usually perform a cystoscopy to make a diagnosis of IC.

The cystoscopy with hydrodistention should be performed under general anesthesia, because the procedure would be too painful for the IC patient otherwise. During the procedure the doctor fills the bladder with sterile water to its capacity and then uses a thin, flexible tube with a light on the end to detect glomerulations (tiny pinpoint hemorrhages) in the bladder wall, inflammation, and/or a thickened and stiff bladder wall.* If a doctor detects Hunner's ulcers, which are open sores, or patches of well defined inflammation in the bladder lining, he or she can vaporize them with a laser wand or destroy them with electrical current. Electrical current is sometimes preferable to laser treatment because the laser can scatter and destroy healthy tissue. A bladder biopsy is also usually taken at the time of the cystoscopy to rule out cancer and reinforce the diagnosis of IC. Some doctors take additional biopsies and use specialized culture methods to detect bacterial DNA in urinary bladder tissue. According to Domingue and Ghoniem, antibiotic therapy is sometimes prescribed when bacteria is present. A non-invasive diagnostic marker for IC based on a noncatherized urine specimen may soon be available. *See What Causes IC.*

When a physician cannot find signs of IC in the bladder, IC is diagnosed by the process of exclusion and patient history. Patients who suffer with bladder symptoms of IC but do not show visible glomerulations during cystoscopy must have some course of treatment regardless of the cystoscopic diagnosis.

* *According to Messy and Stamey visible glomerulations do not appear in the normal bladder, (however) glomerulations are not specific for IC.*

What are the Standard Treatments for IC?

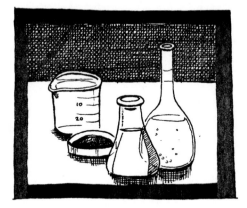

Although researchers continue to search for a cure, there are several treatments available. A new patient who is experiencing bladder pain will often be prescribed a medication to relieve symptoms and pain until one of the standard treatments is established. Even though none of the following treatments are 100% effective, they do offer relief from some of the symptoms and help most IC patients lead a fuller life. However, each IC patient is unique and treatment is very individual. The following information has been gathered from research, IC literature and the individual experiences of IC patients. Many treatments are exclusive to the bladder and don't address IC as a systemic disease. *For more information about treatments or treatment options, contact the ICA or the IC Network.*

Hydrodistention
The diagnostic cystoscopy with hydrodistention is considered the initial treatment for IC, because stretching the bladder wall with water is thought to destroy some of the nerve endings and bladder surface, help break down scar tissue, increase bladder capacity, and reduce urgency and frequency. Patients experience

a temporary worsening of symptoms for a few days after the procedure and prescription medication is necessary. Although hydrodistention is a helpful treatment for many patients, not all patients respond. Many patients who experience relief with the initial diagnostic procedure would not choose to repeat hydrodistention.

Elmiron

The FDA approved drug Elmiron (pentosan polysulfate sodium) is the first oral treatment developed for IC. It works by creating a false GAG layer (the mucous coating of the bladder lining) to prevent leaks into the lining where sensitive nerves are embedded. Although Elmiron can be instilled directly into the bladder, it must be done at least every day so it is prescribed as an oral medication.

Elmiron successfully decreases frequency and pain in a large percentage of patients. The chief side effect of Elmiron is diarrhea which is believed to affect only a small percentage of people. However, Elmiron may be problematic for patients with irritable bowel syndrome (IBS), stomach ulcers and other gastrointestinal problems. Also a small percentage of patients have experienced hair loss and bleeding disorders (it is advisable to discontinue Elmiron three months before surgery).

Some patients may need to take Elmiron in conjunction with another medication, such as Neurontin. Neurontin is a drug used to treat seizures and appears to be helpful in blocking painful nerve impulses in some IC and FMS patients.

DMSO (RIMSO-50)

Bladder instillations are considered the most direct method to treat inflammation. The instillation of a solution containing the anti-inflammatory DMSO (dimethylsulfoxide) via catheter is a standard treatment for IC. The properties of DMSO have analgesic and antihistamine effects and encourage muscle relaxation.

DMSO is helpful to both the ulcerous (Hunner's ulcer) and the non-ulcerous forms of IC and according to LaRock and Sant has a 50% to 90% success rate with non-ulcerous IC and a 50% to 70% improvement rate in ulcerous IC.

DMSO has been on the fringe of medically accepted arthritis treatments for years and was the first drug approved for the treatment of IC. DMSO instillations are absorbed into the bloodstream through the mucous membrane lining of the bladder. Patients experience a garlic-like taste and breath, and sometimes flu-like symptoms, and/or a worsening of symptoms up to a day or two after treatment. Uncomfortable symptoms are thought to be caused by a temporary histamine release from mast cells and chemical burn. Although there have been no serious side effects reported, patients are recommended to have periodic ophthalmologic slit-lamp examinations, blood counts, and kidney and liver function tests a few times a year.

Most doctors believe that DMSO should not be held more than 15 minutes per treatment because a longer "dwell time" may damage tissue and/or deliver systemic absorption. However, the man who pioneered the use of DMSO therapy, Dr. Stanley Jacob, surgeon and researcher at the Oregon Health Science University, believes that IC is a systemic disorder and if a patient is comfortable, the longer DMSO is held in the bladder the better. Dr. Jacob's program for IC includes intravenous (IV) and oral DMSO with upwards to a 90% success rate. Dr. Jacob uses DMSO in conjunction with DMSO2 which contains extra oxygen. DMSO2 reduces the garlic-like odor experienced with straight DMSO. It also appears to help patients with allergies and other conditions when taken orally. Dr. Jacob encourages his patients to use self-catheterization for faster results.*

Typically, doctors give DMSO instillations every one to two weeks for about six to eight weeks. Experts, such as Sant believe that treatments should not begin for about three to four weeks after the cystoscopy when bladder biopsy sites have healed, and if possible, that patients should begin with plain DMSO. Other solutions such as hydrocortisone, lidocaine (an anesthetic) and heparin (a blood thinner) can be added to the DMSO to further soothe inflammation and help repair the bladder lining. Patients who are helped by DMSO usually notice improvement about a month after a full cycle of treatments and return for further treatments as needed. Patients who have difficulty getting to a doctor's office sometimes use self-catheterization, however, urine should be tested to rule out a urinary tract infection (UTI) before an instillation.

Other bladder instillations used for IC include Chlorpactin (oxychlorosene sodium) which must be administered under anesthesia (it is too painful while awake) and usually creates a flare-up before relief, silver nitrate and the experimental medication bacillus Calmette-Guerin (BCG). BCG, a vaccine made of a weakened strain of tuberculosis bacteria, is used to treat bladder cancer by stimulating the immune system. BCG has a high rate of improvement in IC patients. *See Resources at the end of this chapter for more information.*

Bladder analgesics such as marcaine or lidocaine are sometimes instilled alone, as is heparin. The newer bladder instillation Cystistat, (hyaluronic acid) developed to temporarily replenish the GAG layer, is currently being researched. Cystistat is supposed to be held in the bladder at least 30 minutes once a week for four weeks, and then monthly. The success and reaction to this treatment are not yet clear. Like other solutions, it may help some, and worsen or have no effect on other people. Some patients have reported that Cystistat may not burn while being held in the bladder, but may trigger pain after voiding the medication. Results are always individual. Cystistat must be ordered from the Canadian manufacturer Bioniche, through a urologist or treating physician. The company offers refunds to patients who do not experience improvement. *Refer to Resources for more information.*

* DMSO$_2$ bladder instillations may cause more painful symptoms than plain DMSO.

Tricyclic Antidepressants
The tricyclic antidepressant amitriptyline (Elavil) is often prescribed in low doses for pain syndromes (low dose antidepressants prescribed to reduce pain do not affect one's mood or depression). Many IC patients have benefited from its analgesic and antihistamine actions, as well as its sedative effects. As a matter of fact, amitriptyline is made of five medications which appear to help with the different symptoms of IC. Amitriptyline is recommended to be taken at bedtime when it helps to combat nocturia, however, a small percentage of patients prefer to take it earlier in the evening for two reasons. The first reason is because amitriptyline can have a temporary stimulating effect before a sedating one, and the second reason being that the drowsy effects can sometimes last through the next morning if taken too late the night before.

The usual side effects include dry mouth, constipation, dry skin, sun sensitivity, and weight gain. Amitriptyline can be formulated into a topical medication which may be helpful for patients who experience difficulty taking oral medications. However, the oral medication may be more effective. *See Chapter Five for more information.*

Amitriptyline is also used to treat IBS, migraine headaches and FMS. For patients who cannot tolerate amitriptyline, other tricyclic antidepressants such as doxepin (Sinequan), nortriptyline (Pamelor), and imipramine (Tofranil) can be used. Newer antidepressants, such as Prozac or Zoloft, are sometimes prescribed to treat IC pain, but they are not reported to reduce frequency or treat all of the symptoms that the tricyclic antidepressants do.

Hydroxyzine

The antihistamine hydroxyzine (Atarax or Vistaril) is used to block mast cell secretion which stimulates swelling in the tissues of the bladder. This antihistamine works well to decrease pain and frequency because it counteracts allergic reactions and helps to block the neurotransmitter acetylcholine. Hydroxyzine is thought to be most effective after taking it for a few months and also helps patients with allergies, migraines and IBS. Because of its sedating effects, it is best taken at night.

Some patients benefit from the antihistamine and stomach acid-blocker cimetidine (Tagamet). However, there are IC patients who have reported that cimetidine aggravates their bladder symptoms. Over-the-counter Benadryl is an antihistamine that helps some patients, especially to aid sleep. IC patients should not take antihistamines that contain decongestants unless they experience no bladder symptoms with decongestants.

The side effects of antihistamines are most usually dry mouth and drowsiness, although patients may feel stimulated by their effects.

Electrical Nerve Stimulation

- TENS Unit - A TENS (transcutaneous electrical nerve stimulation) unit can be placed above the bladder or on the lower back to help control IC pain. Daily treatments with this non-drug approach work by supplying a mild electrical current that appears to stimulate hormones that block pain, increase blood flow to the bladder and strengthen the pelvic muscles. Relief is cumulative and appears a few weeks to a month after initial use. Usually TENS is not prescribed until other methods of treatment have been tried, however TENS seems to be quite helpful to patients with Hunner's ulcers. The side effects of TENS may include skin irritation and chemical sensitivity.

- <u>Vaginal or Anal Probe</u> - Another variation of TENS used to control pain and frequency is transvaginal or anal stimulation. A device called the Physiostim is a probe that is placed in the vagina in women and in the anus in men. The probe is hooked up to a biofeedback monitor and delivers a low-grade electrical current to block neural pain messages and re-train bladder muscles to hold urine longer. The therapy lasts about 20 minutes and is usually prescribed twice a week for a month. After this period a patient can take the monitor home for self-treatment.

    A patient should find a comfortable body position for inserting and retaining the probe during treatment. Feeling uncomfortable pressure is a signal to reduce stimulation. IC patients should not perform Kegel exercises during treatment. Patients who cannot use a tampon, perform Kegel exercises, or have sexual intercourse without pain, are usually not good candidates for this type of therapy.

    The probe is mainly used to treat incontinence but has helped some patients with pelvic floor dysfunction (PFD), vulvodynia, and IC to strengthen muscles and reduce hyper-activity.

- <u>InterStim Therapy</u> - This newer therapy involves a small neurostimulator which is surgically implanted under the skin of the abdomen in order to generate mild pulses to the sacral nerves (which affect bladder function). InterStim has been used successfully for the treatment of severe incontinence and is gaining attention for its treatment of IC symptoms. Possible side effects include abdominal pain, infection, lead migration and possible sensitivity to the implant (which contains silicone).

- <u>Stoller Afferent Nerve Stimulation (SANS)</u> - The SANS device involves an electrical generator, a cable and a needle which stimulate sacral nerves to suppress overactivity, restore normal bladder function and treat pelvic pain. SANS is not an implant. During a 30 minute session, performed once a week for 10 weeks, a needle is inserted near the medial tibial malleolus (near the ankle). If the procedure is successful, frequency of treatment may be altered. The SANS device helps to treat urgency, frequency and pelvic pain. SANS is not yet approved for sale in the United States.

Pain Medications
Frequency, pressure and pain can demand immediate treatment. Smooth muscle relaxants such as Ditropan and Urispas are often prescribed to stop bladder contractions, help to control frequency and urgency, and help to increase bladder capacity. Drugs that act as bladder analgesics, which include Urised, Pyridium, and over-the-counter Uristat and Azo-Standard are also used to relieve symptoms. Although the side effects of these medications can discourage long term use, they may act as reliable standbys for flare-ups.

On occasion, an IC patient must use stronger medication to treat bladder pain. For example, a patient may need to take a pain medication such as Percocet or codeine to calm bladder pain after a medical procedure, or to break the cycle of an acute flare-up, or when she/he is in pain and cannot take the time from work to rest and recover. However, when a patient cannot break a cycle, experiences chronic, severe pain day after day, has exhausted all other treatments, and can no longer normally function, a pain specialist may be needed.

Doctors who specialize in chronic pain management have discovered that chronic pain patients do not experience the "high" and craving of a drug addict. Although the body can develop a natural tolerance to a drug, a patient who is severely disabled by daily pain may be helped by taking a small, steady, slow release of pain medication through a localized patch, pump or oral dose. This type of therapeutic pain treatment must be monitored closely because there is often a fine line between pain control that can improve the quality of life, and the side effects of pain medication that can interfere with the quality of life. Each IC patient presents individual needs and challenges to the doctor.

Most IC patients do not have to choose therapeutic pain treatment. Fortunately new pain medications with less side effects are becoming available. And as new treatments for IC are becoming available, as well as a better understanding of how medications help to control symptoms, doctors and patients have a better chance of treating IC without narcotic drugs.

Bladder Surgery

Severe and unremitting pain may lead to bladder surgery. Surgery, however, is considered a last resort reserved for only the most severe cases of IC. Surgery may be necessary when pain and frequency become unbearable, the bladder is scarred, stiff and diminished in size, and has a limited capacity to hold urine.

After surgery, some IC patients do feel better, but different types of surgeries offer different results. IC patients still stand the chance of continued pain if the bladder neck, trigone (base of the bladder where there is a concentration of nerves), and urethra are left in place. Patients may suffer from chronic bladder and kidney infections, become incontinent or require self-catheterization due to urinary retention. They may also experience small bowel obstruction or spontaneous rupture with an intestinal pouch (*refer to the next page)*. According to Hohenfillner, Linn, Hampel, and Thuroff (1997, p. 223), "Tragic outcomes of highly invasive surgical approaches to interstitial cystitis have been observed."

- Augmentation - According to the NIDDK, this procedure makes the bladder larger, most often by adding a section of the patient's small intestine, a tube-like structure that absorbs and transports nutrients from food for use by the body. With this treatment, scarred, ulcerated and inflamed sections of the patient's bladder are removed, leaving only healthy tissue and the base of the bladder. A piece of the patient's small intestine is removed, reshaped, and attached to what remains of the bladder. After the incisions heal, the patient may be able to void normally. Even in carefully selected patients - those with small, contracted bladders - the pain, frequency, and urgency may remain or return after surgery and the patient may have additional problems with infections in the new bladder and difficulty absorbing nutrients from the shortened intestine. Some patients are incontinent while others cannot void at all and must insert a catheter into the urethra to empty urine from the bladder.

- <u>Bladder Removal</u> (Cystectomy) - Different methods can be used to reroute urine once the bladder has been removed. In most cases, the ureters are attached to a piece of bowel that opens onto the skin of the abdomen, called a stoma. Urine empties through the stoma into a bag outside the body. This procedure is called a urostomy. Some urologists are using a technique that also requires a stoma but allows urine to be stored in a pouch inside the abdomen. At intervals throughout the day, the patient puts a catheter into the stoma and empties the pouch. Patients with either type of urostomy must use very clean, or sterile steps to prevent infections in and around the stoma.

    With a third method, a new bladder is made from a piece of the patient's bowel (large intestine) and attached to the urethra in place of the removed bladder. After a time of healing, the patient may be able to empty the bladder by voiding at scheduled times or may insert a catheter into the urethra. Few surgeons have the special training and expertise needed to perform this procedure.

Overlapping Symptoms and Conditions

Many IC patients and doctors feel that IC is more than a bladder disease. IC often appears as a multi-faceted disease that affects the whole person. The connection of the overlapping symptoms and conditions is not yet clear and once again many IC patients must find the right doctor to treat another condition or two along with their IC.

It's not unusual for IC symptoms to occur in conjunction with FMS, which like IC, appears to be a disease of neuro-hormonal abnormalities and multiple causes. FMS causes fatigue, stiffness, fragmented sleep, skin rashes, inability to concentrate, sub-normal body temperature, headaches and sensitivity to cold and/or heat, and affects the muscles, tendons and ligaments. FMS also appears to be genetic and is accompanied by other conditions and symptoms. Chronic fatigue syndrome (CFS) is believed by some researchers to be the same illness as FMS. Although a diagnosis of IC does not indicate a diagnosis of another condition, IC patients, especially those who have FMS may experience the following conditions and symptoms: irritable bowel syndrome (IBS), sometimes referred to as a spastic colon; vulvodynia, a condition which causes vulvar pain and inflammation; hypothyroidism, which is a low functioning thyroid; pernicious anemia, a vitamin B-12 deficiency; Sjögren's syndrome, an autoimmune disorder which causes dry mouth, eyes, skin and vaginal tissue, and can affect the connective tissue; mitral valve prolapse (MVP), a faulty heart valve, which sometimes causes a heart murmur and may be related to bladder problems; multiple chemical sensitivity (MCS), which results in sinus and respiratory problems, migraines, numbness and tingling, skin rashes, heart palpitations, dizziness, and sensitivities to an array of chemicals, scents and fumes. A small population of IC patients have systemic lupus or multiple sclerosis.

Symptoms of accompanying conditions are often treated with the same approach used to control the symptoms of IC.

Gentle exercise may be recommended to relieve pain patterns and stress. Hands-on body therapies may be used to release tension and re-educate muscles. Antidepressants may be prescribed to block pain and improve sleep. Antihistamines may be used to calm and prevent symptoms. Following a diet for IC may also help to prevent the symptoms of other conditions.

Many of the conditions that overlap IC are either dismissed or are newly recognized like IC. Although doctors may have biased opinions about these illnesses and the connections between them, some urologists and researchers have taken these connections seriously for some time. Dr. Daniel Claw of Georgetown University Medical Center in Washington, D.C., was quoted in a 1994 ICA Update, "IC patients and their doctors have long speculated about the connections between IC and certain systemic diseases" (p.7). Urologist Kristine Whitmore wrote about the striking similarities IC has with other diseases in which inflammatory processes predominate in her book, *Overcoming Bladder Disorders*. Dr. Stanley Jacob has treated IC as a systemic disorder for decades.

While IC patients network and researchers continue to investigate, the connecting thread of other illnesses is becoming more evident. What cannot be overlooked is the fact that these illnesses mostly affect women. For this reason alone, ***Patient to Patient: Managing Interstitial Cystitis and Overlapping Conditions*** refers mainly to women although many of the treatments and self-help strategies are useful to both sexes.

RESOURCES

Bacillus Calmette Guerin
Ken Peters, M.D.,
Beaumont Hospital,
Royal Oak, MI
www.ic-network.com/chat/chatarchives/peters.html

Bioniche
1-800-567-2028
www.bioniche.com/cystista.html

Dr. Stanley Jacob
(503) 494-8474
www.dmso.org
jacobs@ohsu.edu

Fibromyalgia Network
P.O. Box 31750
Tucson, AZ 85751-1750
1-800-853-2929
fmnetter@msn.com or www.fmetnews.com

National Chronic Fatigue Syndrome and
Fibromyalgia Association
P.O. Box 18426
Kansas City, MO 64133-8426
(816) 931-4777

Multiple Chemical Sensitivities Chemical Injury
Information Network
P.O. Box 301
White Sulphur Springs, MT 59645-0301
(406) 547-2255

National Vulvodynia Association
P.O. Box 19288
Sarasota, FL 34276-2288
(941) 927-8503
www.nva.org

The Vulvar Pain Foundation
P.O. Box Drawer 177
Graham, NC 27253
(336) 226-0704
www.vulvarpainfoundation.org/index.html

National Sjögren's Syndrome Association
1-800-395-NSSA (6672)
www.sjogrens.org

Chapter 2
FOLLOWING A DIET FOR IC

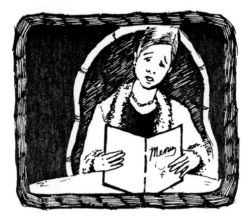

The idea that diet has an effect on the IC patient's bladder remains controversial. Not every doctor nor every patient believes that diet has an impact. Others debate the degree to which diet has an effect. But for the majority of IC patients who experience burning, spasms and frequency after eating certain foods, the need to follow a restricted diet is obvious.

Until recently there has been little research on the relationship between diet and the urinary tract. However, over the last decade several lists of foods to avoid have been developed for IC patients. These lists of foods are all similar in that they exclude spicy, acidic and aged foods, artificial sweeteners, flavor enhancers, and some preservatives and dyes.

IC patient Bev Laumann explains in her book, *A Taste of the Good Life: A Cookbook for an Interstitial Cystitis Diet*, how certain foods send messages within the nervous system and trigger IC symptoms. These foods contain the monamines tyramine and histamine, as well as the amino acids tyrosine, tryptophan and phenylalanine. New research has shown

27

tyramine and histamine to be the most irritating offenders. Foods containing these different compounds are also known to trigger pain in patients with other pain syndromes, such as irritable bowel syndrome (IBS) and migraine headaches. To determine which foods if any irritate your bladder, refer to the following lists. If your bladder symptoms calm down after a few days, introduce ONE food at a time. This process of elimination will help you determine foods to avoid or eliminate from your diet.

Group 1 Foods (Foods To Be Avoided)
aged cheeses (i.e., cheddar, Roquefort, brie)
aged, processed, cured, & smoked meats and fish (or any animal
   product with nitrates)
anchovies
apples
apricots
aspartame (i.e., Nutrasweet)
avocados
bananas
beer
berries (except blueberries and blackberries)
caffeine
cantaloupes
carbonated drinks
caviar
cherries (sweet and sour)
chicken livers
chocolate
citric acid
citrus fruit and citrus juices
coffee
corned beef
cranberries and cranberry juice
fava beans

Group 1 Foods (Foods To Be Avoided) (continued)
grapes
hot spices (those include cayenne, chiles and chile powder,
  cloves, cumin, curry powder, fenugreek, & paprika)
lima beans
mayonnaise
miso
MSG (monosodium glutamate)
nectarines
peaches
pineapples
plums
pomegranates
raw globe or green onions
red wine
rhubarb
rye and sourdough bread
saccharine
salad dressing (commercially prepared)
sodium benzoate or potassium benzoate
soy sauce (except some low-sodium)
strawberries
tea
tofu
tomatoes
vinegar
white wine and other alcoholic beverages when not cooked
yogurt

Group 2 Foods (Limited-Use Foods That May Be Bladder-Safe When Used In Small Amounts)
cooking sherry
cooked globe onions, cooked green onions, raw chives in very
  small amounts
low-sodium soy sauce

nuts (other than almonds, pine nuts, and cashews)
preservatives and artificial ingredients
ripe blackberries
bananas
white chocolate
dried cranberries
raisins
herb teas *
yogurt (Some IC patients say they can eat frozen yogurt.)

Giving up favorite foods may feel like you're giving up little parts of yourself. There's a saying, "You can't let go until you find a replacement." Although there are alternatives and substitutes, each patient has a unique tolerance for different foods. Trying a new food, even if it is considered "safe," may not work for you. A new IC patient just discovering her or his diet restrictions may have to learn through "trial by error." Therefore, using moderation and limiting new foods to times when your bladder symptoms are stable is not only essential to avoid a flare-up, but also necessary to distinguish if a food is really an irritant.

Occasionally patients who have been on an IC diet for a good period of time and have been treated for symptoms, discover they can tolerate foods which they could not before. This can also work in reverse. Sometimes a food that has been completely safe can all of a sudden become irritating to the bladder. Reintroducing it later may work out or the food may always have to be avoided. The bladder can change and the body's chemistry can change. IC is full of surprises, for better or worse. Taking control of your diet can help to reduce the unwanted surprises.

The following dietary alternatives and suggestions have been collected from the broad and individual experiences of many different IC patients. They should be tried in moderation, one food at a time when bladder symptoms are stable. For more suggestions, substitutions and recipes refer to *A Taste of the Good Life: A Cookbook for an Interstitial Cystitis Diet.*

* *Many herbal teas are irritating to the IC patient's bladder.*

Fruit

Most IC patients find canned pears (avoid pears packed in artificial sweetener) to be the most bladder-safe fruit. Unfortunately pears are among foods found to be highly affected by pesticides. To avoid neurotoxic pesticide residue buy organic pears and pear juice.

IC patients may want to try filtered pear juice from the health food store and/or pear juice made for babies such as Gerber's. Pear juice, if tolerable, can add a lot of flavor to cooked dishes, however it may be necessary to dilute it with water. (IC patients should avoid pear juice that contains citric acid.)

Some IC patients find they can tolerate watermelon, blueberries or blackberries, but these fruits are not bladder-safe for everyone. Minute Maid's reduced-acid Orange Juice may be agreeable, as well.

Tomatoes are usually irritating to the IC bladder. For some patients even yellow tomatoes and creoles (true creole tomatoes are only grown in Louisiana) are not safe. Patients who can tolerate tomatoes may do best with the hothouse variety and not the commercial tomatoes from large groceries. Tomato pastes, sauces and juices often contain citric acid which is a bladder irritant; but there are brands that do not add citric acid to their ingredients. For example, Ragu makes a spaghetti sauce without this preservative. Adding a teaspoon of Ragu sauce to certain dishes can provide tomato flavor. This includes chicken or beef broth for IC patients who miss canned tomato soup, which usually contains citric acid and must be avoided. Soups and cereals found at health food stores should also be checked for added fruit juice.

Coffee and Tea

IC patients who can drink coffee, either with caffeine or decaffeinated may want to try a dark roast. Dark roast coffee beans are the lowest in acid. Check with a coffee supplier for acid levels. Patients who drink decaffeinated coffee should make sure the caffeine is removed by a pure water process.

Tea is also acidic. Some patients find low acid coffee more bladder-safe than tea. To be on the cautious side when trying a new tea, dunk the tea bag or tea ball only once in the water.

Sensitive patients will be able to determine if a tea will be agreeable. If a tea passes the bladder test only a few dunks should be used before drinking. Weak tea is usually essential to avoid symptoms. Water should never be poured over a tea bag unless patients are not sensitive. This also applies to herbal teas.

Herbal teas offer many benefits, but some are very powerful, acidic, and contain various medicinal properties. Different herbal teas have different effects. They can act as diuretics, astringents, antispasmodics, sedatives, stimulants, antiseptics, expectorants, laxatives, and more. Although a good percentage of IC patients cannot tolerate herbal teas or must drink very weak tea, one doctor specializing in herbs created a custom tea to relieve IC symptoms. The tea is made from 12 different herbs. Many of these herbs when used alone cannot be tolerated by IC patients. And, although the formula was proven to help a number of IC patients who were in a study conducted by Dr. Kristine Whitmore, Dr. David Gordon, and Dr. Ching-Yao Shi, there have not been good outcomes reported by other IC patients.

Sensitive patients may not be candidates for experimentation. The tea for IC is expensive, and even if one does not show an intolerance right away there may be a cumulative effect on symptoms. Patients should stay on the safe side when first experimenting with this tea. They should use one dunk of the tea bag, take one sip of the tea and then wait 20 minutes (if possible) to void to determine its effects. *

For current information on herbs and their therapeutic effects, as well as their side effects, refer to the book, *The Honest Herbal* by Varro Tyler. *See Chapter Five for more information on the alternative uses of herbal teas. To order Dr. Ching-Yao Shi's tea see Resources on the last page of this chapter.*

* Some patients may feel symptoms much sooner and therefore must empty their bladders sooner.

Sweets and Sodas

Caramel and carob seem to replace chocolate for many patients. Chocolate can be very hard to give up and white chocolate does not have the same effect. However, white chocolate can be satisfying when served hot or added to desserts. The Vermont Country Store carries both vanilla powder to use in place of extract, and a hot vanilla drink to replace hot chocolate. *Refer to Resources.*

Patients who can eat sugar may want to add a little honey to the sweet side of their diet. Honey is a prime source of mineral salts and offers many nutritive benefits (honey should come from a well-known source). However, honey can be strong, so it is necessary to try only a small amount when first testing and keep in mind that there are many different varieties to choose from. Some IC patients are also able to use maple syrup for sweetening and flavor. (IC patients who are prone to yeast infections should limit the amount of sweets in their diets.)

Carbonation in water, soda water and commercial sodas is typically irritating to the bladder and can cause frequency. Patients who can tolerate sodas can let them go flat or add a little salt to get rid of the bubbles. Some patients find Coca-Cola to be the least irritating soda because it does not contain citrus.

Other patients find they can drink 7-Up because it does not contain caffeine and other ingredients found in Coca-Cola. And, of course, there are many IC patients who must avoid all sodas.

Salad Dressings, Condiments, and Seasonings

Eating fresh vegetables is very important, but salad dressings contain a number of bladder irritants. Replace dressings with olive oil and add some mild dry herbs for flavor and nutrients. Olive oil with salt, pepper (some IC patients must avoid ground black pepper) and a dash of oregano is wonderful on salad. Garlic powder, salt, pepper, and oregano mixed with olive oil and a touch of honey (if tolerated) also make a good salad dressing.

Greek olives cured only in salt brine are very flavorful and can help to provide the sour taste associated with the vinegar in salad dressings. Some patients also find that they can eat a small amount of Hellmann's Real Mayonnaise or Miracle Whip. A small amount of either of these condiments can be added to olive oil for flavor in salads or sandwiches. Patients who cannot tolerate mayonnaise products can try softened cream cheese (including the lower fat variety), or butter flavored with herbs.

Try different oils to put more flavor and nutrition into your diet. A small amount of toasted sesame oil and/or sesame seeds can add a lot of flavor to rice and egg dishes. Mirin, a cultured sweet rice flavoring found in health food stores also adds flavor to rice, pasta and dips. Because it is cultured, it may not be bladder-safe for everyone, but a little bit goes a long way and some IC patients seem fine with it.

Dried herbs such as dill, thyme, basil, marjoram, oregano, bay leaf, parsley, rosemary, sage, and celery salt should be tried one at a time to determine which can be used. If tolerated, herbs can offer important antioxidant properties. Garlic and onions also offer healthful benefits as well as flavor to foods. Cooked garlic and garlic powder appear to be tolerated by many patients. (IC patients worried about the strong garlic odor after DMSO may want to treat "like with like." Everyone in the household has a garlicky meal the day of the treatment.) Raw garlic, however, may be too strong. Raw onions, including green onions, do not seem to be easily tolerated either. Patients should be careful to avoid raw onions in salads. Cooked onions are often bladder-safe in small amounts, but onion powder may be an irritant.

Spicy foods should usually be avoided because they stimulate histamine release. However, those who seem to tolerate and enjoy some spicy foods may benefit from trying favorite spices one at a time when symptoms are stable. Highly seasoned dishes often contain an array of spices which can irritate the IC bladder and make it impossible to determine the culprits that might be triggering symptoms.

Peppers, like wines, can vary. For example, a small amount of mild paprika may irritate the bladder while a small amount of fine black pepper may be benign. Paprika is added for color in many foods including hot dogs and sausage. It is also in many hamburger and hot dog buns. Of course, not every IC patient has a reaction to paprika or can tolerate black pepper. All IC patients should use gloves when cutting hot peppers or dealing with other spicy foods, because the juice from hot foods can linger.

Some patients can tolerate spices when they are cooked in food, and some patients find that certain combinations of foods make a difference. Over time, which includes stable time (when the bladder is calm), the IC patient learns what does and what does not work. Unfortunately, it's often by accident.

Cheese

Aged cheeses can be very irritating to the IC bladder, but there are alternatives to fill in their places. Processed cheese such as American Cheese seems to be tolerable, but may not seem so healthy for those who are used to healthy foods. Mozzarella and Ricotta are usually tolerated, however, it's necessary to check different brands to see if vinegar has been added. Fresh goat cheese, which is healthy, is usually tolerable. And, a small amount of American Cheese can add color and flavor to mozzarella, fresh goat cheese or feta (goat cheese in salt brine). Both feta and mozzarella are wonderful in salads, especially with Greek olives cured only in salt brine. Plain processed Parmesan Cheese in a can is also versatile and sometimes tolerated. However, there are IC patients who cannot eat it or they find that the amount eaten makes a difference. (IC patients prone to yeast infections should limit their amount of dairy intake.)

Patients sensitive to salt may need to avoid foods high in sodium. Bev Laumann has found that salt can be good, bad or have no effect on the IC bladder. Several different situations appear to determine the effects of salt in the individual patient. These include daily water consumption, how much the IC patient exercises, whether the IC patient has mostly frequency or pain, if the IC patient has sodium sensitive high blood pressure, and if chlorine in water affects the patient's bladder. *See Chapter Six*. Another problem with salty foods may in fact be monosodium glutamate or sodium metabisulfite which are added to many snack foods that are labeled with "natural flavoring."

Alcohol

Alcohol in general is a bladder irritant, but some patients find they can drink a sweet, low acid late harvest dessert wine such as Sauternes, Barsac or Johannisberg Riesling. A small number of patients have found they can drink a well filtered vodka. And, some say they can drink straight whiskey, even though whiskey is high in histamine. Alcohol and mixed drinks made with tonic, fruit juice or soda can irritate the bladder and usually must be avoided. Plain water and ice (watch out for water and ice made from strongly chlorinated water) are the most bladder-proof mixers.

When drinking alcohol, be sure to do so early in the evening, because alcohol before or near bedtime can interfere with deep sleep (repair time). Alcohol may also increase symptoms in patients with other conditions such as fibromyalgia (FMS) and multiple chemical sensitivity (MCS). Patients taking medication should use caution, following labels and instructions.

Using Prevention and Assertiveness
The following suggestions can help to make life more comfortable, normal and productive:

- LEARN TO READ LABELS to avoid irritating ingredients such as citric or ascorbic acid and vinegar, which is added to many breads. IC patients can have reactions in their bladders to preservatives, natural and not, as well as food dyes. Elizabeth Lee Vliet, M.D., author of *Screaming To Be Heard*, explains in her book how certain dyes in foods (and medicines) act as bladder irritants.
- LEARN TO QUESTION wait staff in restaurants. Call ahead if you are not sure of the food served in a particular restaurant. Most restaurants offer plain (not marinated) steak, chicken and a baked potato. Find restaurants where you can enjoy a bladder-safe meal and where you are comfortable. Be aware that favorite foods some chain restaurants sell in groceries differ, because of the added preservatives used for shelf life.
  If you're invited to a dinner party, if possible, call the hostess or host well in advance to ask what foods will be served. Gently explain that you have food intolerance because of a medical condition. Ask if it's possible to plan a plate for yourself in order to avoid drawing attention to a problem. If this is not possible, and it is a casual affair ask if you can bring your own dish to add to the party. Naturally, there will be times when this will not be possible and

you will either have to decline or pretend - which is often impossible.

- EXPLAIN TO YOUR DOCTORS that you must follow a diet similar to a patient who takes MAO inhibitors and also has a gastric ulcer. Patients taking MAO inhibitors, which are a class of antidepressant drugs, must avoid foods or beverages that contain tyramine.

- EAT REGULARLY to prevent flare-ups. Eating small amounts of food throughout the day is very therapeutic for the bladder. This can also be helpful to patients with IBS and migraine headaches.

  Patients who suffer from constipation should be sure to eat first thing in the morning to stimulate bowel activity. A bowl of hot oatmeal or oat bran eaten between dinner and bedtime can also add to stimulation the next morning. Protein for breakfast is important for stamina and fresh vegetables should be substituted for the lack of fruit in a diet for IC.

- AVOID DEHYDRATION to avoid IC symptoms. Dr. Lowell Parsons, Professor of Urology, University of California, San Diego, noted in a 1993 *ICA Update* that, "70% of the IC population have a leaky bladder lining." (p.2-3) He explained how these leaks allow salts (Dr. Parsons has studied the effects of salt on the IC bladder) and other substances to diffuse through the lining and into the bladder wall and cause symptoms. Dr. Parsons expressed that, "patients suffering with leaky bladders who drink less fluid have more concentrated urine and more symptoms and pain so they tend to drink more water to dilute their urine. In contrast, patients without leaky bladders tend to drink less water so they do not have to urinate frequently." Other theories on the effects of salt in the IC bladder have been proposed.

- DRINKING WATER VARIES. Tap water can trigger symptoms due to high levels of chlorine and other harsh chemicals. Some patients benefit from using a water filter and some patients prefer to use a water filter for cooking and use bottled water for drinking.

Filtered tap water also exposes IC patients to various chemicals, and bottled water may be an irritant to some IC patients. Bottled water is usually disinfected with ozone and a small number of people, especially those with an auto-immune disease, cannot tolerate ozone. Ozone can be detected with O_3 paper from a lab supply company. It also can be removed from water by boiling or exposing it to air. Imported bottled water such as Evian has a long shelf life and, therefore, is usually free of ozone.

IC patients who experience problems with bottled water may need to drink distilled water instead. Distilled water is the safest for the sensitive IC patient, but a patient who can drink bottled water may benefit. Distilled water can flush important minerals from your body and should be avoided when ill or dehydrated. Reserving distilled water for flare-ups or alternating it with compatible bottled water may be best.

- PAY ATTENTION TO YOUR HORMONAL CYCLE, because bladder pain and frequency can fluctuate with a woman's menstrual cycle. It's important to recognize foods that may be more tolerable during the different times of the menstrual cycle.

    Some women with IC discover that they can cheat on their IC diet when their estrogen level is highest, because estrogen helps with the formation of the protective layer of the bladder surface. However, other IC patients find that when their estrogen levels are highest they suffer with IC symptoms because of the stimulation of mast cell secretion in the bladder.

- NEUTRALIZE ACIDIC FOODS with the dietary supplement Prelief. Prelief has been helpful to some patients when they are experiencing burning symptoms. It has also helped patients to tolerate a number of foods. A study conducted by Dr. Kristine Whitmore showed that many IC patients could tolerate acidic foods and drinks, such as tomato sauce and alcohol, when Prelief was taken before or consumed with foods or drinks. (Prelief can also be used as a calcium-source supplement.)

Prelief, Tums, baking soda, Tagamet, and Zantac can be used to neutralize acidic urine, however, patients should consult their doctors before trying these products and medications. They may react unfavorably with medications and/or be dangerous for patients with certain medical conditions. *See Resources.*

- CONSULTING A NUTRITIONIST OR DIETITIAN is helpful if she or he understands IC. Patients working with a dietitian or a nutritionist initially should bring along a copy of a diet for IC. "Dietary professionals are used to building their patients' immune systems with fruit juices, fortified foods and vitamins," explains a Philadelphia dietitian who is experienced with IC. "However, with a diet for IC, most patients have an opportunity to reduce the inflammatory process in their bladders and, therefore, improve their health." She continues, "Because IC patients are all so different, it can be difficult to determine irritants. Some patients experience pain and frequency soon after their saliva mixes with the juices of an irritant. Others may have a hard time pinpointing the culprit. I suggest using a litmus to measure the Ph balance of the urine."

  "I also advise my patients to eat small meals frequently and also sometimes suggest acupuncture or acupressure to strengthen the immune system.* There is a real need for research in alternative therapies, but what works can depend on the disease process in the individual."

- BE AWARE THAT REACTIONS TO VITAMINS AND SUPPLEMENTS aren't well documented. Like a diet for IC, advice and information should be referred to as a suggested guideline. Also, like trying different foods, patients may need to use caution when trying supplements. IC patients can experience pain and spasms when their bodies cannot properly metabolize the breakdown of different vitamin supplements. Supplements may also be problematic because of their "inert ingredients" (fillers and binders).

- Knowledgeable urologists suggest that IC patients avoid vitamin C (ascorbic acid) that has not been buffered with calcium carbonate. Sometimes they suggest patients try "ester C." Many IC patients find that vitamin C causes burning and spasms even when it is buffered. When a patient cannot take vitamin C she or he must try to replace this important antioxidant by eating broccoli, green, red and yellow peppers, Brussel sprouts, dark leafy vegetables, cabbage, potatoes and watermelon (if tolerated).

Many IC patients have difficulty taking B vitamin supplements, especially B-6. However, most patients find vitamin B-6 tolerable in foods such as fish and whole grains (watch out for rye). Although some patients find they can tolerate an individual B supplement such as B-1 or B-12 (which is fermented and may cause problems), IC patients should be sure to add many of the following B-rich foods to their diets: liver (chicken liver may trigger IC symptoms), salmon, tuna, eggs, beef, oysters, pork, milk, mushrooms, broccoli, spinach, dried beans, enriched breads and cereals, brown or enriched rice, and other enriched flour products (if tolerated).

Dietary supplements are currently very popular and appear to be helping many people to cope with common conditions. However, IC patients must be very cautious when trying different supplements, because many will trigger bladder symptoms and other reactions. IC patients often cannot tolerate the natural supplements suggested for their FMS, chronic fatigue syndrome (CFS) or other conditions, although a few supplements have actually been found to be helpful in treating IC symptoms. One is the amino acid L-arginine which appears to be most helpful to patients who have larger bladder capacities or those with a history of bladder infections before IC. L-arginine must be pure and is preferably purchased through the company Biotec (*See Resources*). Another supplement some patients have found helpful for treatment of IC symptoms is Algonot, a combination of chondroitin and glucosamine sulfates. The GAG layer, the mucous lining of the bladder, is made of glycosaminoglycan. More information is needed on this supplement, but it has helped patients with FMS and arthritis, as well as IBS. (Some people cannot tolerate chondroitin.) IC patients who are interested in trying different supplements should contact the IC Network or the ICA for studies, information and patient experience. *See Resources in Chapter One.*

Whether you can take vitamins and other supplements or not, it is essential to eat foods that supply generous amounts of vitamins, minerals and protein. Taking charge of eating habits can help to ensure nutritional needs, and prevent painful symptoms.

Experts disagree as to whether the IC patient's immune system should be boosted or not.

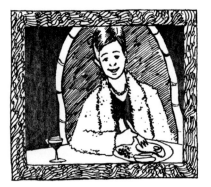

Children with IC and Diet

Parents need to give their child with IC a lot of support, especially regarding diet restrictions. Parents must be willing to research which foods to avoid, experiment with their child's diet and learn to be very creative. Children usually like the challenge of trying delicious new recipes, eating healthy foods (including fruits and vegetables not treated with pesticides) and learning to read labels. Children are also motivated to learn when they feel special. Parents can reinforce a child who is trying a diet for IC by taking an interest. Educating family members, the child's school and the parents of her or his friends are also important.

The most difficult foods for children to exclude are popular snack foods and sweets, especially those containing citric acid. Referring to Laumann's recipes can be a big help. Older children may feel resentful, but if certain foods cause them to have painful symptoms, they will most likely decide to avoid these foods. However, there are more issues to deal with for a teen with IC. Sometimes a good social worker can help.

RESOURCES

COOK BOOK
A Taste of the Good Life:
A Cookbook for an Interstitial Cystitis Diet
B. Laumann
(This book offers IC patients much more than recipes.)
Order from the IC Network or the ICA
Refer to Laumann's column "Fresh Tastes" featured once a month on the IC Network website. *See Resources in Chapter One.*

PRODUCTS
Dr. Ching-Yao Shi's Chinese Herbal Tea for IC patients
1-800-558-9833
www.easternherb.com

L-arginine
Biotec
1-800-345-1199

Prelief
AkPharma
1-800-994-4711
www.prelief.com
(Free samples and information available through AkPharma. Prelief can also be found in grocery and drug stores.)

The Vermont Country Store
(802) 362-8440
www.vermontcountrystore.com

The Pain Pattern of IC

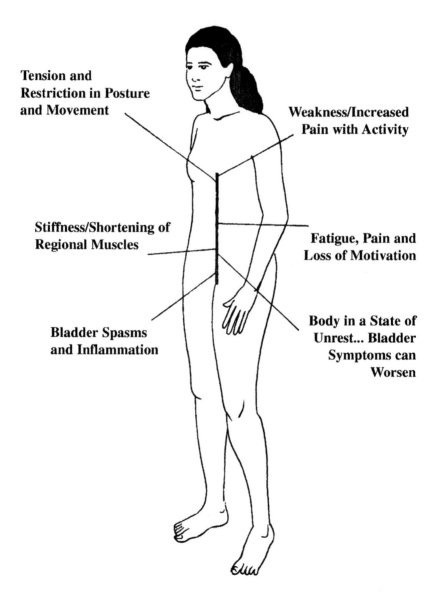

Tension and
Restriction in Posture
and Movement

Weakness/Increased
Pain with Activity

Stiffness/Shortening of
Regional Muscles

Fatigue, Pain and
Loss of Motivation

Bladder Spasms
and Inflammation

Body in a State of
Unrest... Bladder
Symptoms can
Worsen

Chapter 3

RECLAIMING COMFORT
IN YOUR BODY

Proper support, good body mechanics and the right kind of gentle exercise can help reduce unnecessary tension. When your body loses its natural resilience and strength from an ongoing inflammatory process such as interstitial cystitis, everyday activities can become a challenge. Even sitting in any one position or on the wrong surface for too long can increase tension and pain.

PROPER SUPPORT FOR YOUR BODY

Sitting

When you are sitting, your pelvis and lower back become the natural base of support for your upper body. If your base of support is weakened by an inflammatory process, you usually will have to overuse other muscle groups such as your abdominal and hip flexor muscles (front of the hips) to comfortably maintain a sitting position. This compensation increases when you add upper body movements such as typing and desk work. If you sit for a living, use a supportive chair, stretch your upper body a little before standing up and get up often and move around.

For many IC patients sitting comfortably means sitting with their hips slightly rolled back and under. In this position both the lower and upper back should be supported with pillows or cushions. Bending your knees and elevating your feet on a foot rest can take even more pressure off your pelvic floor by allowing the abdominal and hip flexor muscles to rest. If you need to work in bed, use an elevated bed tray as a laptop desk. No matter what position you sit in, it is essential that you find proper support and that you change your position periodically.

Standing

When you are standing your feet become your base of support. If your hip flexor and hamstring muscles (the large muscles in the backs of your legs) are short, tight and weak, your body's weight will have a tendency to rest back into your heels. In this posture, walking can cause a jarring impact to your pelvic floor, and forward movement, such as walking and climbing stairs, becomes dependent on already tightened hip flexors. The ICA Self-help brochure recommends that the IC patient consider wearing a shoe with a soft rubbery sole and a slanted heel as well as foam inserts for additional cushioning. With this in mind, you should remember to avoid wearing shoes with a negative heel (a heel that is lower than the toe of the shoe which is the case in some sandals), or a high cut over the instep.

If you spend a lot of time at home you should also pay attention to the shoes or slippers that you wear around the house. Slippers generally do not offer much support for your feet or body when you stand or walk, so be sure to add foam inserts for extra padding.

Lying Down

Your whole body is supported when you are lying down. Unfortunately, night can be the most uncomfortable time for patients with urinary frequency. Not only is it tiring getting in and out of bed to use the bathroom, but it is also difficult to let your body relax when you have a constant awareness of your bladder and the other muscles in that area. You can benefit from sleeping in a bed that is not too hard, so muscles can rest comfortably and "let go." However, it's also important for patients to avoid a bed that is too soft and/or uneven, so muscles won't have to work to find the right support needed for relaxation. If you sleep with a pillow between your knees, you should use a small baby pillow instead of a standard size, which can put pressure on your hips. Sleeping is repair time and it is important to get as much quality sleep as needed.

Good Body Mechanics

Start each day by warming your spinal muscles and disks before getting out of bed. To do so, sit up on the side of the bed before standing. Place your feet comfortably apart on the floor. Bend your elbows and touch your finger tips. Imagine that your forearms are resting on an imaginary shelf. Relax your shoulders and very gently rotate your upper body side to side. Lead the movement with your eyes so that your head turns first. Be careful not to arch your lower back. Begin with three gentle rotations every morning before standing. Work your way up to a comfortable amount.

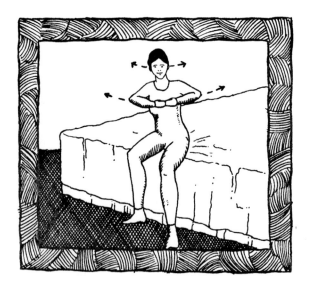

Since the bladder is most active in the morning and early hours of the day, IC patients should be cautious not to physically overextend themselves during this time. Stressing stiff and weak muscles can lead to uneven tone and the inability for muscles to find a normal resting position after use. IC patients should also avoid overstretching their muscles and learn to use their legs for proper support when bending and lifting. If the low back and hips are especially tight and weak, bringing the knees together before bending forward or lifting can provide extra support and stability. Ideally, it's important to strengthen the leg and gluteal (buttocks) muscles to help with everyday movements.

Objects should be carried close to the body with both arms and should not be very heavy, otherwise lifting may result in tiny tears in the muscle cells. These tears often occur when a person engages in eccentric movement, which involves contracting or working a muscle while moving the ends of the muscle further apart. In other words, stretching a muscle while also contracting or using it. Lifting heavy dishes out of the dishwasher and vacuuming the floor are good examples of this type of muscle work. Keep challenging chores such as vacuuming and unloading the dishwasher to a minimal time limit. Break up your physical work. Learn to problem-solve, use proper body mechanics, keep physical goals realistic, and maintain your strength.

Use A Conservative Approach To Exercise

Exercise can be a beneficial ingredient to pain management. Exercise encourages deep breathing and circulation, helps with digestion and elimination, therefore, reducing both physical and mental stress. If you are successfully practicing a regular workout routine, don't stop! If you are experiencing fatigue, muscle and joint pain, and/or IC symptoms after any physical activity, you need to consider the value of gentle exercise.

Proper stretching, strengthening and some moderate aerobic activity are necessary to release the muscular restrictions that accompany IC. It is essential to continually encourage range of motion, flexion and extension of the spine, length in the muscles, as well as strengthen the lower and upper back to prevent spasms and joint pain. For optimum relief, a suitable exercise routine should be practiced three to four times a week and be combined with intermittent stretching daily.

Some options for gentle aerobic activity include water exercise and regular walking. If you choose an upper body workout in water, make sure that the water is warm and over your shoulders. Although your heart gets a better workout in waist deep water, the high water level will help to support your upper body. *To find a water workout class, information on Water Walking and/or alternatives to chlorine and bromine refer to Resources on the last page of this chapter.*

If walking is your goal, find a complementary warm-up routine that offers gentle stretching, plus a few strengthening movements designed to promote even tone in your body. To determine what a gentle warm-up routine feels like, try the exercises on the following pages:

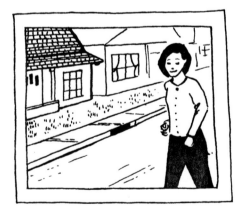

The Full Body Stretch

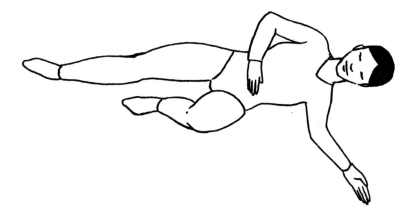

Lie on your back on a comfortable surface. Extend your opposite arm and leg. Take a full breath, and then slowly exhale as you let your back relax into the floor, bed, etc. Repeat by exchanging your arms and legs.

- Keep your shoulders relaxed and your extended arm comfortably bent.
- Make sure that your chin is not tucked under.

Knee/Chest Rock

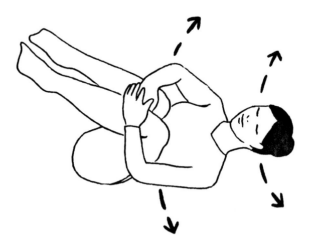

After you have completed **The Full Body Stretch** bring your knees toward your chest, one at a time. Lightly hug your knees with your arms, and then gently rock your body side to side. Let your eyes lead the movement so that your head turns first.

- Avoid locking your fingers too tightly while hugging your legs.
- Keep your shoulders relaxed.

Strengthening Your Back

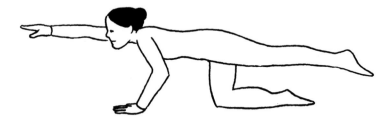

Roll over onto the easiest side and get up onto your hands and knees. Position yourself on all fours, then lift your opposite arm and leg long enough to find your balance. Release, look down and repeat this exercise by exchanging your arms and legs.

- Avoid lifting your arms and legs higher than your spine.
- Keep your shoulders down and avoid straightening your lifted arm.

The best motivation for movement is the reward of feeling better. If you are able to attend an exercise class be sure the movements are fairly unchallenging. You should minimize eccentric and repetitive movements, as well as avoid holding one position or stretch for too long, which is often required in most warm-up sessions. To prevent triggering pain, you may also want to avoid machines that impose strenuous postures, and repetitive, or imposed movements (e.g., ski machines, stair climbing machines and treadmills). Even the pushing leg movements of bicycling may add to the pain pattern of IC.

If you try to follow an exercise video, limit the amount of repetitions of each given exercise, as well as the time you hold any stretching position. Walking in place can substitute unwanted repetitions and performing other stretches can fill in time during long held positions. *Refer to the IC Stretch/Exercise Video for stretching and toning options. See Resources.* The video can be ordered from the ICA. Preference and capability for exercise is, of course, very individual and even more so for the IC patient.

If you experience sore, stiff and tight areas after gentle exercise, use ice. In time these areas should improve with the right type of exercise, or the exercise should be avoided. Never continue a movement that causes pain. The philosophy of "working through the pain" will only tighten up tense areas and create more problems. Reach your goals realistically and realize that there will be times you will not be able to exercise. Take advantage of the good days to keep up your strength, but also remember to be careful not to overdo!

RESOURCES

Aquatic Exercise Association
1-888-AEA-WAVE (232-9283)

The United States Water Fitness Association
P. O. Box 3279
Boynton Beach, FL 33424-3279
(561) 732-9908

IC Stretch/Exercise Video
Interstitial Cystitis Association
(301) 610-5300
1-800-ICA-1626 (422-1626)
www.ichelp.org

Chapter 4

TRYING HANDS-ON, TRADITIONAL & ALTERNATIVE THERAPIES

Most interstitial cystitis patients initially seek help from urologists for relief of their symptoms. Typically, the first interventions that IC patients receive are treatments and medications for the bladder which have been empirically shown to relieve IC symptoms. However, these traditional healthcare approaches do not always alleviate IC symptoms. Some patients subsequently seek help and pain management from an array of traditional and alternative healthcare professionals other than urologists in their search to relieve and control the accompanying symptoms and conditions of the illness.

During the past few decades a holistic awareness has evolved about mind/body interactions which affect the treatment of chronic illnesses. Today, courses in alternative medicine are offered to medical students, nurses, physical and occupational therapists, and social workers. Wellness and prevention programs are now covered and encouraged by many insurance and managed care companies. Pain management programs are increasingly available in hospitals and physical therapy clinics.

Many doctors who treat newly researched illnesses are grateful to have more to offer their patients. These physicians are most likely to be receptive to alternative treatments and often feel that IC is more than just a bladder disease. They also believe that there are therapies besides bladder treatments and medications which have the ability to address the whole person.

Alternative healthcare approaches are helpful for treatment of the overlapping conditions of IC, but like some traditional treatments, they are often ineffective in alleviating bladder symptoms. No one treatment, whether alternative or traditional, works for all IC patients. Genetics, pre-existing injuries and illnesses, personal lifestyles, beliefs, and the treatment, or lack of treatment from healthcare providers can affect the success of any IC intervention. The receptiveness of patients to new treatments is often related to the severity of their bladder symptoms. Patients with less sensitive bladders may be more willing to explore a variety of therapies. In contrast, individuals with more sensitive bladders face the possibility that new treatments will fail and actually aggravate symptoms. These patients will naturally be more hesitant to try new interventions after having had too many bad experiences.

Many healthcare professionals do not understand IC and are not flexible enough to listen closely to the unique needs of IC patients. This lack of understanding can leave patients feeling alone when they seek help away from their urologists. In addition, there are far too many healthcare practitioners who in turn, blame IC patients when there is no improvement from therapies. It is not unusual for alternative practitioners to have been trained to believe that the patient is 90% responsible for the outcome of the therapy, and the practitioner responsible for 10%! This thinking has quietly come to be known as "new age guilt."

A good therapist or healthcare practitioner will never promise that they can cure you, and will accept the fact that you have a physical illness that is very difficult to treat. In particular, any new age cure-all treatment should be viewed with skepticism because of unrealistic claims.

Mind/Body Medicine

When holistic medicine (treatment for the whole body) caught on in the 1970's, the students and followers were mostly young and healthy when they embraced the preventive lifestyle to avoid illness. Like other young people at that time they were very idealistic about their studies and practices. Many took pride in avoiding the field of traditional medicine.

The roots of alternative medicine lie mostly in ancient Eastern methods of healing and prevention, as well as European behavioral theories, and mentalist philosophies handed down from the latter 19th century and early 20th century before the organic nature of many illnesses was recognized. Alternative pioneers carefully broke down many Eastern theories and approaches to health, then reinterpreted and blended these ideas to our Western way of thinking.

Problems and illnesses in the different organs and parts of the body were considered as psychological in nature and "stress" was recognized as the cause of disease instead of the trigger for disease. For instance, during the 70's an alternative practitioner may have believed that a nearsighted person's eye difficulties were caused by a trauma during childhood. According to this belief, the trauma would have prevented the eye muscles from developing normally because the child had withdrawn his or her vision, become introverted or too shy to want to see. Misunderstood illnesses affecting women were also labeled as stress disorders. Endometriosis was called the "working woman's disease" and believed to occur in "type A" personalities (overachievers). Somatization disorders were considered to be physical disorders caused by emotional conflicts, anxiety and depression which the patient could not confront. Consequently, it was believed that these disorders became unconsciously displaced onto the body, or into the body parts.

Although stress should not be underestimated in its ability to make us susceptible to illness (stress may cause histamine release in the bladder), it was misunderstood and misconstrued as it worked its way into the psycho-babble of the 70's. The blaming in the 70's was not limited to the field of alternative medicine. During this time medical students were still being taught that IC and many other conditions mostly affecting women were of a psychological nature. Treating the mind was extremely popular. While the holistic, or mind/body field, embraced many wonderful treatments and techniques to heal the whole body, Western medical doctors were experimenting with new philosophies and new drugs to treat the mind.

Today mind/body medicine has become more sophisticated. Alternative practitioners and teachers have aged and lost some of their idealistic views. Traditional doctors have become more open minded to chronic pain conditions. Diseases and diagnoses are now better understood by both fields and harmful beliefs have come a long way from the days when multiple sclerosis was called "faker's disease." As East really begins to meet West some very wonderful and important techniques from both fields of medicine are being utilized for their powerful benefits. Many different therapies are available to help patients recognize, reduce and manage the ongoing stress of chronic illness. However, each chronic pain patient must be realistic about the "just do it" philosophy of today's world. For this reason the therapist should be considered as important as the therapy itself. Appropriate therapy also depends on the individual. The following information is intended to offer insight into various modalities and how they may or may not be beneficial to IC patients.

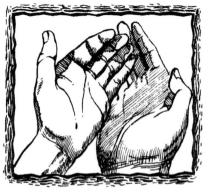

Massage

The goal of massage is to increase circulation, reintroduce a feeling of well-being, and recreate a sense of relaxation and comfort that may be lost in the pain cycle of IC. A good massage therapist will be able to facilitate these improvements by loosening tight muscles, encouraging flexibility and increasing a cooperation of body parts.

A good massage therapist will take a history of your symptoms, check with you often about the comfort of your position, and the amount of pressure and strokes used during the massage session. Like too many repetitious movements performed during exercise, too many repetitious strokes to one area of the body during a massage session can cause additional tension in a patient with chronic pain. Massage strokes should be firm (not hard) and smooth. The room temperature should be comfortable. A good rule of thumb to follow when working with a therapist is that *if it feels wrong, then it is wrong for you!* Doctors, physical therapists, chiropractors, and reputable massage schools can usually recommend a good licensed massage therapist. Be sure to ask for someone who has had experience working with chronic pain patients.

Myofascial Therapies

Many different myofascial techniques are available today. Although physical therapists will probably use soft tissue mobilization, students of physical therapy are now studying various techniques. Some therapists combine techniques and others are very disciplined in one modality or theory.

So called "bodywork" is not new and has been well developed during the last quarter of the 20th century. One popular technique, used by a number of IC patients is myofascial release, which focuses on releasing the fascia, the supportive connective tissue surrounding the muscles. Another manual therapy that has proven to work well for both fibromyalgia (FMS) and IC patients is Aston-Patterning. This multifaceted work integrates myo-kinetics, which addresses restrictions in soft tissue (fascia, muscles and tendons); arthro-kinetics, which addresses the restrictions around and through the joint tissues; and neuro-kinetics, which addresses movement education, ergonomic and environmental modification.

Practitioners of Aston-Patterning also offer gentle work to release the muscular system of the urogenital diaphragm.* To locate a practitioner specializing in myofascial release contact local physical therapy clinics and massage schools. *See Resources to locate a practitioner specializing in Aston-Patterning.* Although there are a limited number of Aston-Patterning practitioners, you may find a physical therapist with some training in Aston-Patterning. Ask the training center when you call.

IC patients should be very careful to pick muscle therapies that use gentle encouragement to lengthen and unravel tight muscles at the client's or patient's own pace. They should be cautious of therapies that attempt to impose an ideal body type (shape or posture), also. Many practitioners use deep tissue work to realign the body to provide more postural support, however, because there is an ongoing inflammatory process in the bladder it is usually not wise to try to realign the pelvis. Practitioners often must be told this before working.

Deep tissue work should mostly be limited to tightened areas around the joints (direct pressure to the joints should be avoided). Surrounding muscles should be blended with firm and smooth strokes. Deep tissue work can help to break up scar tissue or adhesions, and the referred tension of IC, but may cause too much change for the patient with an inflammatory process in her or his bladder.

When work is too deep or a session is too long, patients may experience spasms and/or exhaustion for a couple of days after, or a new cycle of pain may begin. IC patients often do not have the tone to support their structural muscles and surrounding tissue after they have been released, so they may end up tensing their tightened deep muscles and the corresponding joint areas for strength. As a result, patients may end up with a "rag doll" effect. Also, if one specific area of the body is over-worked or "overly loosened," other muscles can end up in a tight tension pattern in order to compensate for the imbalance.

IC patients should avoid therapies that combine hands-on techniques with psychotherapy during the same session. Such techniques are designed to break emotional holding patterns that have settled in the body. Psychotherapy is best achieved when clients or patients are free to feel emotions at their own comfortable pace. Emotional patterns usually release naturally with proper myofascial therapy. Most massage or myofascial therapists are not licensed or trained in psychotherapy, therefore, this combined technique can be harmful when specific theories are imposed on clients.

* For more information about pelvic therapies see "Medical Diagnosis and Treatment" in Chapter Eight.

Physical Therapy

Physical therapy (PT) is often prescribed for IC patients with persistent muscle problems or a diagnosis of FMS. PT is especially helpful to IC patients who experience limited range of motion, as well as muscle and joint pain. Many IC patients find relief from PT work on the psoas and piriformis muscles, which attach to the hip. A good prescription for PT will include soft tissue mobilization, the myo-therapy most accepted in the medical field. This manipulation focuses on the release of the soft tissues (the fascia which is the connective tissue surrounding the muscles).

A knowledgeable physical therapist will use firm, smooth and blending strokes to encourage even tone, and will help patients or clients to become aware of their own tension patterns and how IC contributes to these patterns. Proper stretching should be introduced before gentle strengthening.

Sports medicine should almost always be avoided. IC patients don't need more physical challenges.

IC patients often need encouragement, which requires a therapist to be more open to the specific limitations of IC. These limitations may include the inability to support small hand weights or find the strength to start the pushing motion of a stationary bicycle without triggering symptoms. Therapists familiar with FMS should be aware that IC patients with FMS may need different treatment than FMS patients without IC. Techniques that are used for FMS, such as "spray and stretch" (used to help muscles loosen and regain range of motion by the use of a cold spray), and "trigger point injections" (injections of an anesthetic into tender point trigger points), may not be helpful to IC patients. Patients who suffer with the overlapping condition of chemical sensitivity may also have a reaction to the spray used in the "spray and stretch" treatment. This is not to dismiss the benefits of muscle pain relief. If general muscle pain is much more persistent than bladder pain, then treating the muscle pain may be more beneficial.

Craniosacral Treatment

This technique is sometimes used by physical therapists, myofascial therapists, and massage therapists. According to the *Fibromyalgia Network Index & Glossary,* Craniosacral treatment is geared towards restoring the proper function of the dural tube. This tube is the connective tissue that lines the inside of the cranium (the head bones), separates the lobes of the brain, and passes down through the foramen magnum (the hole in the base of the skull). The dural tube encases the spinal cord and contains the spinal fluid.

Craniosacral treatment can help to calm bladder symptoms and referred muscle pain when done by an experienced practitioner. As with every modality, this work should begin conservatively.* Since Craniosacral treatment is often combined with other massage techniques, it may be difficult to judge its effectiveness. It may be best to initially experience Craniosacral treatment separately. *See Resources for trained therapists and more information.*

The practitioner should avoid lifting the IC patient's head too far forward while cradling to feel the pulse of the craniosacral system. Traction should be gentle and as brief as possible. Deep work may have to be avoided.

Chiropractic
Good chiropractic care is another approach to relieving muscular and neurological problems. Gentle adjustments to the spine have helped some patients break the pain cycle of IC. An experienced chiropractor will use releasing techniques to relax tight ligaments and muscles around the adjusted joints, as well as, encourage flexion and extension. A full adjustment may have to be broken up into two visits, depending on the tightness of the muscles. Ideally, patients should alternate chiropractic visits with massage sessions. Patients should also practice gentle stretching and toning to keep their spinal alignment.

Acupuncture
Acupuncture is gaining popularity for the treatment of chronic pain. Thin needles are placed in specific areas of the body to encourage the natural flow of energy and restore the immunities that illness has interfered with. Acupuncture helps release endorphins to fight pain and is thought to help the bladder by expanding the blood supply, which increases beneficial oxygen and nutrients. This increase is important for patients with frequency, because the constant voiding decreases the amount of oxygen and nutrients flowing to the bladder.

A conservative approach to acupuncture is essential for IC patients, because the energy released during a session may be too strong and stimulating for those prone to anxiety. Practitioners should be made aware of this problem and avoid beginning with the acupuncture points for the bladder. Practitioners should also be willing to check frequently with their patients during treatment.

To get the best results, acupuncture sessions need to begin on a regular weekly basis. If a patient experiences improvement (it may take several weeks), sessions should be continued periodically for maintenance.

To find a licensed or certified acupuncturist contact a hospital, wellness clinic or school of acupuncture, if available. *To find a member of the American Academy of Medical Acupuncture (an active licensed medical doctor or doctor of osteopathy) see Resources.*

Herbal Medicine

Some acupuncturists, as well as other practitioners, use herbal supplementation to enhance the healing process. Tinctures, teas, tablets, tonics, and sitz baths have long been used for treatment of bladder disorders. Today, there is research to understand how the particular ingredients in herbs work. However, finding the herb which will work for IC patients is still "trial by error" and very individual. Patients with severe pain should understand that herbs cannot mask bladder pain as effectively as prescription drugs. Patients who are very sensitive to foods and medicines should also know that certain herbs can have an over-relaxing, contracting, burning, or stimulating effect on the bladder. *See Chapter Two and Chapter Six for more information.*

Homeopathy

Homeopathy is another non-drug treatment that uses naturally occurring essences of plant, mineral or animal origin to treat illness and pain. Homeopathy is based on the concept that "like cures like." This concept is the same idea used in allergy and immunization shots. The homeopath, naturopath or other health practitioner administers a small dose of a homeopathic remedy

65

to stimulate the body's natural immune defenses and the healing process.

IC patients who take prescription drugs may benefit from a homeopath who is also a M.D. Homeopaths who are physicians can have a better understanding of the relationship between the patient and the disease, and the role of the patient's prescription medicine. Although homeopathic remedies are sometimes helpful to IC patients, homeopaths often look for a specific emotional event or experience that correlates with the symptoms and onset of their patients' illnesses rather than simply focusing on the physical aspects of the disease.

Mind/Body and Pain Management Programs

Mind/body and pain management programs are designed to help chronic pain patients with coping strategies, such as relaxation and guided imagery, cognitive restructuring (modifying one's response to her/his painful and troublesome symptoms), behavior therapy, practical lifestyle modifications, group therapy, exercise, and sometimes nutrition management. These programs are designed to empower individuals and provide them with a feeling of control and success. Within each program there are usually a number of patients with different chronic conditions or symptoms. Because each participating patient brings a unique set of symptoms, emotions and abilities, it is necessary for all patients to feel the support and understanding of the facilitator.

Although most patients are encouraged to participate at their own pace, IC patients might need to make modifications for their specific needs. The following suggestions may be helpful and some can be used in place of the instructed methods:

- MODIFICATIONS FOR COMFORT - When you begin a program let your facilitator know if you have frequency, and need to sit near a door to leave without interruption. Bring a cushion for sitting or back support. You will usually be given the option to bend your knees when lying down.

- MODIFICATIONS FOR EXERCISE - Use your own judgment when asked to take certain positions or perform certain exercises. The positions and slow motions in movement rituals such as yoga or Tai Chi may be too demanding, however a facilitator will usually offer alternative options for individual needs. If you need to sit out of an exercise, try to do so without interrupting, and then talk to your facilitator after class about your future needs unless you are instructed differently.

- NUTRITION MANAGEMENT - Eating is thought to release endorphins which make us feel better. Learning good nutrition and how foods can help to fight pain is very important, however, some foods such as those that elevate serotonin levels can cause bladder pain and frequency in IC patients. *Refer to Chapter Two for nutrition information.*

- BREATHING MODIFICATIONS – Techniques such as mindful breathing use diaphragmatic breathing, which focuses on movement in the belly. Diaphragmatic breathing is very important to IC patients because they often do not breathe fully due to pain. However, not all IC patients can comfortably focus on their bellies without setting off bladder pain or frequency. Instead, IC patients can produce the same helpful results by focusing their breath into their ribs.

To begin this breathing exercise, place your hands on your lower ribs and rest your elbows out to your sides. Now gently breathe in and imagine your lower rib cage (front, back and sides) expand and become wider, so you are aware of the three dimensional movement of your whole rib cage. On your exhale, picture your ribs resting down and coming closer together. As you continue this exercise, gradually move your hands and breath up your rib cage so you feel the movement under your arms and across your shoulders. Make sure that your inhale is gentle and not forced, and that you use a long and slow exhale. This style of breathing will encourage a natural response of movement in your belly without stirring the inflammation in your bladder. Be sure to take a few moments before standing after this exercise.

Relaxation Exercises

Relaxation, or guided imagery exercises that require patients to focus on their sites of pain in order to relax, or imagine the healing process taking place are not usually as successful as distraction exercises for IC patients. Instead of focusing on the bladder, IC patients can try focusing on one hand to achieve relaxation. However, reintroducing movement and feeling to other areas of the body that are tense and painful because of referred IC pain may help.

When techniques and relaxation exercises are used to decrease the stress and fears that accompany the pain of IC, they can help to calm and control the illness. Practicing relaxation daily encourages the healing process in both the body and mind. One wonderful stress management technique is called Focusing. It is especially helpful to deal with worries or problems that don't seem manageable. With regular practice, relief is experienced in the body. It is best to begin with the instruction of someone else's voice.

Focusing

Start by closing your eyes. Take a few cleansing breaths and imagine that you are stepping back from your problems for awhile.

- Now picture a place like a beach or park, a beautiful and comfortable place in nature, a place that feels safe. Wherever it is, it is a place where you will be able to empty your bladder comfortably if needed. You are in total control.

Find a comfortable place to sit and take in the beauty of this place.

• Sense the temperature, the smells, the sounds of the birds, the wind in the trees or the surf. You feel very peaceful in this special place. Allow yourself to take it all in with no pressures to do anything or go anywhere.

• After you feel the comfort and serenity of this place see if there is an issue or problem that has been in your way. If there is more than one problem pick the biggest. Don't let yourself think about it, just pick it out.

• Now take this problem or a few problems if you cannot choose one, and place them away from you on a far rock, hill or tree top.

• After you place your problem or line up your problems on a distant site, notice what comes into your feelings. Notice if there is anything else, maybe something that you did not consider as the problem right away or something that you didn't consider so important. If there is something else, line it up on the distant site. Take a breath and make a choice, pick one issue, one that feels right or stands out for now.

• After you have done this take a few cleansing breaths and notice how you feel with your problem so far away. Now picture yourself standing up, turning, and walking away, leaving the rock, hill or tree top behind you. As you turn and walk away take in the beauty of this very special place.

• When you are ready slowly open your eyes and take a little time to stretch and focus your eyes. Now notice how you feel. Perhaps you feel lighter, more relaxed and have a different perspective than before this wonderful exercise.

Post Traumatic Stress Syndrome

Although it is beneficial to learn how to cognitively deal with a flare-up (modifying the response to pain to better cope with the situation), the pain of IC automatically induces an emotional response. Many theorists, both traditional and alternative, believe that chronic pain patients often can't cope well with their pain because it brings up old traumas and unsafe feelings. In some instances this is true. For many IC patients the trauma of past negative, painful and unproductive doctor visits and procedures have resulted in some post traumatic stress. Nevertheless, the unique pain of IC causes behavior that is often misunderstood and mislabeled even by pain management facilitators who claim they are experienced and familiar with the disease.

IC patient Naomi McCormick, Ph.D., and pain specialist Daniel Brookoff, M.D., understand the pain of IC. In a joint article in an early 90's ICA Update, McCormick expressed, "It is nearly impossible for an IC patient to be emotionally neutral about pain." The pain of IC is carried to the center of the brain that carries emotion, and because IC affects an internal organ (the bladder), it is considered visceral pain. Visceral pain sends messages to the part of the brain called the limbic system which regulates arousal and emotion. The messages from the bladder pain can make a patient feel upset, emotional and depressed as a result. Dr. Brookoff specializes in chronic conditions that cause severe pain and are not easily treated or understood. He helps many IC patients with pain management.

Unfortunately, the type of behavior that IC pain sets off is similar to the type of behavior seen in patients with post traumatic stress syndrome, especially those who have been sexually abused. IC patients may be seen as emotionally laden victims of a traumatic experience demonstrating hyper-vigiliant behavior (the need to be on guard against harm), instead of a person in need of medication to treat the unsettling symptoms of interstitial cystitis. Because many IC patients are unable to sit still, relax or focus on their bladder pain, they may be misjudged. It is important for patients to discuss this issue with a pain management program facilitator to avoid being misunderstood.

Compulsions, quirks or eccentric behaviors that exist before IC will stand a chance of being magnified during flare-ups. And, it is not unusual for IC patients to experience their first symptoms of IC after a stressful event. Stress does not in itself cause IC. Jay A. Goldstein, M.D., (1996) described how patients (with FMS and chronic fatigue syndrome) are born with a genetic blueprint. He explained that genetically predisposed individuals may be "overtaxed" and "depleted" of important neuro-hormonal transmitting substances. Goldstein believes that "this might explain why most patients develop their illness during situations of increased environmental stressors of various types" (p. 7). These individuals may not have what it takes chemically to fight infections, over-exertion and trauma.

Many practitioners in both the alternative and traditional field continue to be guilty of misdiagnosing chronic pain patients as victims of stress. And when these patients do not get proper medical treatment, they can suffer and display enormous stress from being placed in this misfortunate situation. An unproductive, vicious cycle often results because these patients have been diagnosed and judged incorrectly.

RESOURCES

Aston-Patterning Training Center
P.O. Box 3568
Incline Village, NV 89450
(775) 831-8228

Upledger Institute
(Craniosacral treatment)
11211 Prosperity Farms Rd.
D325 Palm Beach Gardens, FL 33410
1-800-233-5880

American Academy of Medical Acupuncture
(Patient referral line)
1-800-521-2262

Chapter 5
COPING WITH NEW PRESCRIPTIONS, DOCTORS & SENSITIVITIES TO MEDICATIONS

As with different foods, certain medications can trigger interstitial cystitis symptoms. The idea that different drugs can have such an effect on the bladder is hard for many doctors to accept.

According to an early IC survey, a large percentage of IC patients suffer with sensitivities or severe allergic reactions to medications. Even so, there is little documentation and not much known about the side effects medications and their fillers can produce in IC patients.*

The following is not intended to augment the information given to patients by their own doctors. Instead, it is meant to help chemically sensitive patients find the right doctors, medications, and treatments without side effects.

Doctors usually understand that IC patients must avoid medications that increase serotonin and norepinephrine levels. Tricyclic antidepressants used to treat IC appear to interfere with the actions these neurotransmitters have on the central nervous system.

TRIAL BY ERROR

Dealing with New Doctors
When seeing a new doctor for a problem other than IC, patients don't know if the physician will be receptive to their IC needs. The doctor, after all, is interested in treating the condition for which he or she is being consulted. Bladder disease is not the

doctor's main concern and a patient's knowledge about her or his body may be dismissed. Even when seeking treatment for an overlapping condition, such as fibromyalgia (FMS), a sympathetic specialist familiar with chronic pain patients may not understand or agree with IC pain management. As a matter of fact, doctors who specialize in newly researched diseases often have opinions as to the cause and treatment for conditions that support their theories and specialties.

Feeling challenged in the doctor's office is a normal experience for most women. According to Elizabeth Lee Vliet, M.D., author of, *Screaming To Be Heard*, "All of us as women often encounter a discounting and devaluing of our wisdom about our bodies and our health needs when we walk in the door of most medical offices." Sadly, this circumstance disempowers patients, causes emotional pain and sometimes results in physical pain. IC patients may become so discouraged by such negative experiences that they give up on treatments and medications that may help them. Some patients just settle for pain or other conditions that might be treatable, or relieved by the right doctor who will work with their needs.

Fortunately, there are doctors who evaluate the success of treatments for chronic pain patients differently than for the average population. This is so important to the many IC patients who are sensitive, do not respond quickly to treatments or cannot fit into standard treatment agendas. However, on occasion doctors may choose not to treat sensitive patients in order to avoid hurting them. Or, patients may not get treatment when doctors who do not know how to treat them speak in a clinical manner to hide their ignorance. There are also some doctors who are afraid of being sued by patients who list many allergies and drug sensitivities. It is necessary to understand these dynamics to avoid useless, repeated visits to doctors who cannot help.

Trying a New Prescription

Prescription drugs and their fillers, the inert ingredients in medications, go through the body in different ways. Both synthetic and natural medications can affect different parts of the central nervous system and cause allergic reactions. This is no surprise to the many IC patients who experience drug reactions and sensitivities in their bladders as well as in other areas of their bodies. The side effects to the central nervous system and the atypical reactions of many IC patients make trying a new drug difficult and often frightening.

Consulting a *Physician's Desk Reference* (available at many public libraries), or the *Pharmacy Guide to Over-The-Counter and Natural Remedies*, and/or becoming friendly with a pharmacist can be helpful and sometimes necessary in order to find information about drug fillers used in medications, documented drug interactions and side effects. A knowledgeable pharmacist can also direct the customer to a formulating or compounding pharmacy, which may be able to tailor a prescription to the individual's needs or offer natural sources which may be better tolerated than synthetic ones.* *See Resources at the end of this chapter.* A pharmacist can offer information on alternative options to oral medications, such as topical creams, ointments, skin patches and liquid medications (which often contain less additives). The most valuable information, however, may come from from another IC patient with similar symptoms. It was an IC patient who first alerted a doctor about what hurt her or his bladder. It was a good doctor who researched the reason and informed other patients and doctors.

When unsure of a newly prescribed medication, ask the pharmacist for only three pills to begin with. Explain to your doctor and your pharmacist that you will fill the whole prescription if the medication doesn't set off your IC symptoms or other reactions. If you are very sensitive to medications, you can ask your doctor if it's possible to begin with a quarter or half dose and gradually increase to full dosage. Let your doctor know that you understand the small amount is not enough to treat the condition, but that this is a necessary experiment for your bladder and other sensitivities. If you usually experience a cumulative effect, and don't experience IC symptoms until a few days or weeks after taking a new medication, inform your doctor that you may not know if you can tolerate the medication right away.

Teaching hospitals may have formulating pharmacies for patients.

If You Have a Bad Reaction

Always let a doctor know if a drug has an adverse effect on your bladder or elsewhere. Although you may not want to deal with a doctor after a problem, you give your doctor the false impression that you improved with the prescribed treatment if you do not let him or her know otherwise. The doctor may also possibly make the same mistake with another IC patient.

It is helpful to report adverse drug reactions to the drug companies. Drug companies are not required to list the inactive ingredients in their drugs, but they do have to disclose the ingredients to individuals upon request. They also record adverse reactions.

The IC patient usually isn't a so called "good patient," and some doctors can make the IC patient feel indulgent and neurotic. When this occurs it's best to try to find another doctor. Although it takes time, energy and often courage to regroup before a new doctor search, the IC patient need not continue to be victimized by the disease and the wrong doctor.

Dealing with Serious Conditions

When other conditions are serious they can be hard to treat without disturbing the bladder. Chronic heart conditions, cancer and other life-threatening illnesses require treatments and medications that can interfere with bladder maintenance in IC patients. Some patients would rather avoid a diagnosis or treatment of a serious condition because they are naturally afraid of an adverse reaction in their bladders. Chronic pain patients often become used to feeling lousy or being told that their various aches and pains are probably nothing or just part of their disease, so they end up dismissing their symptoms. Dismissing symptoms can be dangerous to IC patients, especially as they get older, because they may not take the aging process into account. They may not take painful signs seriously, and may back away from doctors and new treatments because they were not helped in the past. IC patients may unconsciously choose to compromise their physical health to avoid physical pain, judgment and dismissal. Because IC patients become wary, they sometimes risk overlooking a serious situation.

As doctors see more IC patients they will recognize IC as more than a bladder disease. And, as patients learn more about the systemic effects and overlapping conditions of IC, they will be able to take better care of themselves. Until this happens IC patients need more self-empowerment and respect from doctors. Both doctors and IC patients need education and encouragement to deal with this complicated disease. It's very important for patients to encourage doctors who show interest and concern for IC patients. It is also important for IC patients to help educate doctors of the IC patient's needs and educational resources.

Surgeries and Hospital Stays

Dealing with surgeries and hospital stays can be very difficult for IC patients. Although it may not always be possible, it's helpful to be fully prepared before going into the hospital for surgery or certain treatments. Preparation is especially important for those who have experienced bad reactions to drugs or those with multiple chemical sensitivity (MCS).

Patients who are undergoing surgery and have the opportunity beforehand should talk to the anesthesiologist about existing drug sensitivities. The doctor may take an interest and work with them individually. Patients who are particularly sensitive to drugs may want to also contact Dr. Ann McCampbell of the Multiple Chemical Sensitivities Task Force of New Mexico. Dr. McCampbell can provide information for sources of preservative-free medications and other products for sensitive patients. *See Resources.*

Although it is helpful to avoid certain medications, it may still be impossible to avoid bladder irritation. Many IC patients have overlapping conditions and require pre-operative medications that can irritate the bladder. Therefore, it is important to plan and consider what pain management can be used after surgery to reduce pain from a procedure as well as pain caused by the adverse effects of medications. Patients should always let doctors know about any additional medications brought to the hospital.

After surgery some IC patients find a morphine shot or drip, or a shot of the anti-inflammatory Toredol effective for pain as well as bladder-safe. Oral Toredol has produced IC symptoms in some patients, but the injection appears to be bladder-safe for others. Patients who use heat or ice for pain may need to order hot or cold packs before surgery.

Since IC patients often experience urinary frequency after surgery, it is important to plan ahead. Depending on a nurse to come in frequently with a bedpan is unrealistic. Plus, bedpans aren't very sturdy and are not meant for constant use. The best solution may be a potty chair placed beside the bed, or patients who do not have adverse reactions to catheters might ask to be catheterized for surgery. This procedure can help rid irritating urine and urgency. However, it's necessary to ask for a pediatric catheter which is smaller and more comfortable. It's also necessary that the nurse knows to check the urine bag often. It may fill up more quickly than the average patient's.

Avoiding air pollution in the hospital room can be another challenge to IC patients in an emergency hospitalization.

Those who are sensitive to odors and fumes can ask in advance, if possible, for a hospital room that has not been newly painted or carpeted, or sprayed with pesticides. While in the hospital, housekeeping can be informed not to use strong disinfectants or cleaning products. If the hospital stay is short it may be best not to have the room cleaned. Strong perfume worn by the caretakers can also be a problem for sensitive patients, but it is not always easy to get people to listen. Wearing a mask when needed may be necessary.

Another very important consideration for IC patients is dietary management. Patients who must follow a diet for IC can talk to the hospital dietitian and plan meals before the hospital stay. It can be difficult or sometimes impossible to get a plain soft boiled egg or a baked potato, because many hospitals contract with outside vendors and have limited internal resources. Arranging to have meals brought in may be necessary. Although a microwave and refrigerator are typically available for patient use, it is unrealistic to expect hospital staff to warm meals or bring snacks. A private sitter or certified nursing assistant may be needed the first day or so.

Coping with General Conditions, Routine Exams and Procedures without the Drugs and Fillers that might Trigger IC Pain

Commonly used medications, as well as certain medical diagnostic exams and routine procedures, can present a challenge to many IC patients. Medications that are used for general conditions may trigger bladder pain. These include acid-blocking and antiulcer medications, antibiotics, anti-inflammatory medications, anti-nausea medications, cough medicines, epinephrine and other decongestants and stimulants, laxatives, muscle relaxants, and stool softeners. Many inactive ingredients in medications can also trigger bladder pain and other sensitivities. Magnesium is one additive that may adversely affect IC patients. Magnesium is used in a number of medications and is known to be a bladder irritant. Another inactive ingredient found in numerous medicines, including tricyclic antidepressants, is silicon dioxide. Although this silicone compound has NOT been proven one way or the other to be harmful, some researchers are taking a closer look at it. *Information on the effects of silicone is presented in Chapter Six.*

IC patients who experience skin rashes and digestive problems with oral antidepressants may be helped by using a formulating pharmacy. One such pharmacy in New England has been working closely with a Boston pain clinic to formulate alternative options for IC patients. These options include antidepressants and pain gels in topical cream forms. Topical medications are often not as effective as oral medication, and usually must be applied a few times a day.

Information and options in this chapter are intended only as suggestions and should be discussed with your doctor.

Dental Visits

An array of different chemicals and materials (including latex or vinyl gloves) are used in the dentist's office. One of the biggest culprits for the IC patient is epinephrine. Epinephrine is used in injections, inhalers, eye drops, and nose drops. Epinephrine is added to the numbing agent in the injection given before an invasive dental procedure. Epinephrine will affect the tone of the bladder and may cause IC symptoms. IC patients can ask the dentist to skip the epinephrine. The numbing agent may be short lived without epinephrine and an additional injection may be required, but this is usually more tolerable than experiencing IC pain during or after a dental procedure. Some IC patients, however, are also sensitive to certain numbing agents. Patient with MCS may experience sensitivity to numbing agents, too. Trying alternative agents may be necessary.

Other substances used during crown work can trigger bladder pain and chemical sensitivity. If you have experienced problems after crown work ask your dentist or surgeon for an ion temporary crown instead of an acrylic one and for non-eugenol cement (made by Proviscell). Let your dentist or surgeon know if glues, astringents or bleaches are irritating so he or she will work closely with you to find alternatives, such as using saline solution instead of bleach when possible. Also ask your dentist or surgeon if you can avoid a medicated pack with your temporary crown. Although an antibacterial agent may be necessary, if it can safely be avoided, you may avoid bladder pain.

IC patients with mitral valve prolapse (MVP) often have another problem when they are advised to take an antibiotic before dental work. Patients who cannot tolerate oral antibiotics without bladder pain may instead try an antibiotic drip before dental work (of course, even some antibiotic drips can affect the bladder). It is very important that IC patients with MVP work closely with primary care doctors. Some patients with very mild MVP are told by doctors that an antibiotic is not necessary and new research from a Framingham Heart Study, which followed 3,500 people, has found not only that mitral valve prolapse was less common than previously believed, but also that most of those who had it were not in jeopardy of the conditions heart-rhythm disturbance, heart failure, stroke, and endocarditis. This information was presented in a 1999 *Harvard Women's Health Watch*. Patients who are interested in discussing this information with their primary care doctor can back order *Harvard Women's Health Watch* volumes. *See Resources in Chapter Eight.*

Dental work can often irritate the bladder no matter how well pain prevention has been practiced. It's also not unusual for some IC patients to experience prolonged pain and inflammation in their teeth after a procedure. This condition, however, does not mean that IC patients should not have the dentist or oral surgeon double-check their dental work.

Eye Exams, Solutions and Drops

Not many patients are aware that what goes into their tear ducts goes into their system. Patients who are sensitive to epinephrine might avoid bladder pain and other reactions by asking their doctors to leave the epinephrine out of the dilating drops used during a routine eye exam. Although the epinephrine enables the drops to last longer, a routine eye exam will usually work fine without the use of epinephrine.

Eye drops in general contain medicines, preservatives and stabilizers that may irritate the IC bladder. Eye medications are often available in both drops and ointments, and ointments seem to be less irritating. However, if drops are necessary Dr. Sidney M. Wolfe, and Rose-Ellen Hope, R.Ph., suggest in their book, *Worst Pills Best Pills*, that a person lie down and apply gentle pressure with the thumb and middle finger to the inside corner of the eye for five minutes after applying each drop. Following these instructions can help to block medications from draining through the duct and decrease side effects. Of course, with any new eye medications it's important to begin with the lowest dose.

Sensitive IC patients who wear contact lens may not realize that contact solution might be a bladder irritant. Even though buffered and preservative free solutions are available, they can contain other irritating ingredients such as boric acid, which some patients cannot tolerate. Experimenting by wearing glasses instead of contacts for a few days may indicate if a solution is triggering IC symptoms. Patients who suffer with dry eyes may find they have a reaction to commercial brands of saline solution. However some patients can tolerate Moisture Eyes by Bausch and Lomb. Alternative brands of eye drops are available at health food stores or shops that sell natural remedies. Some of these brands are homeopathic and a small amount can be very strong and sometimes irritating. To identify which drops are irritating, try brands with the fewest ingredients and use only a small drop in one eye to begin with.

Bronchodilator Inhaler

Inhalers used to treat asthma often contain epinephrine and other stimulating chemicals that can affect bladder function in IC patients, as well as cause other unpleasant reactions in those with chemical sensitivity. IC patients with respiratory problems may have to use a steroid inhaler to avoid bladder spasms. Although inhaled steroids work preventively with long term use and are not intended for the short term treatment of an asthma attack, they can work quickly to reduce histamines in a respiratory response to chemicals and irritants. However, patients with MCS often report difficulty with inhalers. Treatments must be discussed with a doctor, preferably one who understands and believes that sensitivities are real and *organic* (caused by a physiological malfunction).

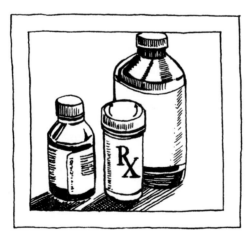

Antibiotics

Probably the most difficult drugs for IC patients are antibiotics. Antibiotic use was once suspected as being a cause of IC. Although this theory is no longer considered valid, many IC patients have taken a lot of antibiotics, and antibiotics often trigger IC flare-ups. Unfortunately, there's not much information available on this problem, and most doctors have difficulty understanding or even treating patients who are sensitive to antibiotics.

The antibiotic ciprofloxacin is sometimes prescribed for patients who are allergic to other antibiotics. This strong antibiotic may or may not be bladder-safe for all IC patients, although there has been speculation that ciprofloxacin might contain pain relieving properties.

If a patient doubts the need for a prescribed antibiotic, the doctor can be asked to check, if possible, to see if there's a bacterial infection. When antibiotics are necessary the doctor should be able to work with a patient to prescribe one that is fairly bladder-safe. However, depending on the infection, at some point an IC patient may require an antibiotic that is irritating. Some patients find that they have less reactions in their bladders when antibiotics are given intravenously (this procedure may not be covered by insurance) or taken in one megadose if possible, but this is not always the case.

Pain medications may be necessary when taking irritating antibiotics. Patients who use antidepressants to treat their IC may find it helpful to take a very small amount of an antidepressant when pain occurs. (Of course, it's necessary to be cautious when taking a drug during the day which is usually intended for use at night.) Another way to fight breakthrough bladder pain is with a prescribed topical pain gel. Although combination pain gels containing more than one medicine are often helpful, IC patients should try one ingredient at a time. For more information contact the New England Compounding Center. *See Resources.*

Antibiotics can set off more than bladder symptoms. They can cause vaginal yeast infections, especially in women with IC and other chronic conditions. Antibiotics can also trigger stomach problems and an array of reactions in sensitive patients.

Preventing Yeast Infections

Both the medication to treat yeast and the yeast infection itself can irritate the bladder, so it's always necessary to use prevention. Only wear 100% cotton panties and change them during the day if they become damp or moist. Use only unscented soaps and detergents. Avoid fabric softeners. Cleanse the vaginal area both morning and night, and change towels daily. Avoid tampons, or use the smallest size and change after each urination. If you are chemically sensitive to the synthetic materials in commercial sanitary pads and tampons, look for natural pads at the health food store or use washable Glad Rags, which are also found at most health food stores. Use an ice pack to sit on while traveling in a hot car, but make sure to remove it as soon as it begins to melt. Wear skirts and don't wear underwear while at home. Always avoid tight pants or synthetic leggings.

Keep sugar and milk intake moderate. Some patients find a diet for IC helpful for fighting yeast, because it eliminates fermented foods. Other patients find a yeast-free diet helpful to prevent both yeast and IC symptoms. Eating a little yogurt daily, if tolerated, may help to prevent vaginal and intestinal imbalance (there is debate among healthcare practitioners as to the effects of eating yogurt). Taking a milk-free acidophilus, which is usually available at both drug stores and health food stores may also be beneficial (*see Treating Yeast Infections*). There are several books available on yeast prevention.

Treating Yeast Infections

Vaginal creams used to treat yeast can create burning and spasms in patients with IC and vulvar vestibulitis. Vaginal creams may contain glycol propylene, alcohol or sulfa which are often irritating to vaginal tissue. Some patients find they can tolerate a small amount at a time, about an inch of cream right before bed. Although this small amount may not work as quickly to cure a yeast infection, it's helpful to those who can tolerate it. However, it's usually necessary for IC patients to keep the medication away from the urethra during insertion. Some find that plastic applicators cause less pulling and are more efficient for delivering medication. Others may find it necessary to use medication only every other night. More than a few tubes of medication may be required to get rid of the infection.

Another treatment option for yeast infections is Diflucan (fluconazole), an oral antifungal prescription drug. This medication is strong and needs to be prescribed and monitored by a doctor. Diflucan is not an optimal treatment for all IC patients, although it seems to be helpful to some patients with IC and vestibulitis who cannot use or get results with vaginal creams. Patients with vestibulitis also sometimes use intravaginal boric acid to treat yeast. Tough to treat yeast infections appear to respond to boric acid, but sensitive IC patients may not tolerate boric acid very well.

Acidophilus can be helpful. Schiff makes a milk-free oral form that some IC patients can tolerate. Itsy Bitsy Acidolphilus made by General Nutrition Center is a baby chewable form that may be bladder-safe and helpful. However, a more direct way to treat vaginal yeast is to insert acidolphilus vaginally, either in capsule form or in powder form inserted with an applicator (available at some health food stores). IC patients should avoid oral acidolphilus that contains aspartame. Patients may also find internal yogurt impossible to use.

The antifungal drug nystatin is sometimes prescribed to treat stubborn yeast infections. This is a strong medication and has been reported to cause bladder symptoms in some IC patients.

Treating Other Vaginal Infections

Bacterial vaginosis can require an antibacterial medicine such as the oral or vaginal cream Flagyl (metronidazole). Flagyl is a very strong drug and many IC patients have reactions in their bladders and elsewhere when they use it. Patients who find this drug intolerable should ask their doctor if they can be treated with the drug Cleocin (clindamycin) instead. Some IC patients seem to be able to tolerate Cleocin better than Flagyl. As always, treatment is very individual so it's best to be on the bladder-safe side and try vaginal creams a little at a time. Vaginal creams are usually better tolerated than vaginal gels which have an alcohol base.

It's essential for IC patients to see a gynecologist when an infection is first suspected. Infections left untreated can become more difficult to treat and sometime require oral antibiotics. Always follow preventive measures.

Treating Stomach Problems

Antiulcer and acid-blocking medications including Tagamet, which is sometimes used to treat IC symptoms, can actually irritate some IC patients' bladders. Suppositories and other medications used to treat nausea are not always bladder-safe, and medications to stop diarrhea can trigger IC symptoms in some patients.

To relieve common nausea without drugs that might interfere with bladder function, try an old-fashioned remedy, Cola Syrup. A small amount mixed with non-carbonated water can help to relieve nausea. Cola Syrup ordered from The Vermont Country Store (*see Resources*) does not contain caffeine and appears to be bladder-safe for some patients. Of course, those who cannot tolerate flat Coca-Cola should not try Cola Syrup.

Other alternative treatments for an unsettled stomach include a weak cup of chamomile, spearmint or peppermint tea. Patients sensitive to herbs can try just one or two dunks of a tea bag or tea ball, and just a few sips of tea. Sometimes this is enough to help settle an upset stomach. IC patients who cannot tolerate peppermint tea may be able to drink spearmint. Plain mint teas are available through Celestial Seasonings found in health food stores and some commercial groceries. (Patients should avoid distilled water when they have diarrhea, flu, are vomiting or when dehydrated.)

Common diarrhea can be relieved with a few sips of slippery elm tea every half hour. Slippery elm soothes the membranes of the intestinal tract. Honey can be added to sweeten the tea. Although slippery elm is usually well tolerated by most IC patients, just two or three dunks of a tea bag or ball should be used. Eating a little barley or oat bran can also help control common diarrhea, however, barley green may irritate the bladder because of its high magnesium content.

Constipation can be somewhat relieved and prevented by using flaxseed or olive oil. Olive oil is usually well tolerated by IC patients, is very healthy and can be used generously on salads or vegetables. Relieving constipation can be very difficult for those with irritable bowel syndrome (IBS), especially during perimenopause. Patients with IBS should consider avoiding wheat and dairy products and follow a diet for IC as prevention. However, patients need foods that supply adequate amounts of B vitamins, because constipation can be caused by a lack of B vitamins. *See Chapter Two for more information on foods and the prevention and treatment of constipation and common diarrhea.*

Laxatives are often irritating to the IC bladder, however, over-the-counter Ducolax seems to be tolerated by some. IC patients should be careful not to become dependent on laxatives or stool softeners. They should also cut back on dairy products when taking laxatives.

Acid reflux is a disorder that can accompany IBS. Reflux can also be caused by certain prescription drugs. Acid-blocking drugs are not always tolerated by IC patients and some patients find brands bought over-the-counter more irritating because of the added preservatives used to further shelf life. Prevention, such as following a diet for IC, avoiding snacks before bedtime and elevating the head of the bed four to six inches is usually the best approach to reduce common acid reflux.

Tums and Prelief can neutralize stomach acids that have an effect on esophageal reflux, as well as neutralize the acidity in the urine of IC patients. IC patients, however, need to let doctors and pharmacists know if they are taking drugs that neutralize acidity, because the ingredients may interfere with the absorption of other drugs, including some of the drugs used to treat IC symptoms. Patients who take Tums are recommended to do so between meals. *For more information or to order Prelief, see Resources in Chapter Two.*

Treating Allergies and Colds

Treating allergies with antihistamines may also help to relieve bladder symptoms. The drug hydroxyzine (Atarax and Vistaril) has actually been proven effective for the treatment of IC, allergies (not colds), migraines, and IBS thanks to the studies and interest of Dr. T. C. Theoharides and Dr. G. R. Sant. *See Treatments in Chapter One for more information.*

Antihistamines that contain decongestants can trigger IC symptoms. Patients who are sensitive to decongestants should avoid nose drops, sprays and pills that contain decongestants. Although some IC patients are able to tolerate small amounts of nasal spray, others find they must treat nasal congestion with steam instead. Steam can actually be very effective when used two to three times a day. The easiest way to steam is to sit on a chair and lean over a sink of hot water with a towel over the head. Drinking hot soups and weak teas (if possible) can also relax and open nasal passages.

Other effective treatments for sinus relief, maintenance and prevention of allergies and colds include nasal rinsing and nasal ointment. Irrigating the nasal passages with baking soda and water can be done with a syringe (ask your pharmacist) or with a Naso Cup. A small amount of the nasal ointment Boroleum can also be swabbed into the nostrils to relieve dry nasal tissue. Both nasal rinsing and Boroleum offer health maintenance with daily use. To order Boroleum call The Vermont Country Store. To order a Naso Cup call Isabella. *See Resources.*

Boroleum is probably not safe for patients with MCS, because it contains camphor and menthol. It also may not be suitable for patients taking a homeopathic remedy.

Patients with chronic sinus problems are sometimes prescribed a steroid nasal spray which is like a steroid inhaler. IC patients seem to be able to tolerate this type of treatment, but it is best to first try prevention by modifying the environment and avoiding fermented foods, sugar and dairy products that increase mucous.

Sore throats and coughs that come with colds and flu can be helped with warm saltwater gargles a few times a day. Antihistamines should be avoided. Popular cough drops may also have to be avoided, because they can set off bladder symptoms. Some patients have found they can tolerate Thayers Slippery Elm Throat Lozenges and Ricola Natural Herb Cough Drops. Look in health food stores if these cough treatments are not found in local drug stores. Always try a new cough drop for only a few seconds. Often a cough drop is not as irritating and still helpful if it isn't finished.

IC patients should be cautious when trying prescription expectorants. The expectorant Humibid has been known to set off IC flare-ups, even when a very small amount is used. The generic form of Humibid, guaifenesin, is sometimes prescribed as a treatment for FMS. FMS patients with an irritable bladder may want to avoid this expectorant.

Certain herbal teas can help to soothe mucous membranes and loosen mucous. However, many of these herbal teas can also irritate the bladder. Safer alternatives include weak tea made from a little dried dill weed. Dill is good for coughs.

Dried sage tea can be used to soothe sore throats. Sage tea can also be used as a gargle. Slippery elm and licorice root teas are very soothing, however, licorice root is strong and not always tolerated by bladder-sensitive patients. All teas should be tried using only one quick dunk of a tea bag or tea ball.

For general aches and pains that come with the flu try plain (weak) chamomile tea. Chamomile is a great relaxant. For prevention of colds and infections try weak tea made of dried thyme. Thyme is also helpful when used in cooked foods and so is garlic, if tolerated.

Treating Migraine Headaches

Migraines, like IC, can be treated with antidepressants and drugs such as hydroxyzine. Other medications such as muscle relaxants and anti-inflammatories may affect the bladder. Drugs that contain a blood vessel constrictor, a sedative or acetaminophen may create bladder pain and frequency. Although beliefs about estrogen and the menstrual cycle vary, some experts believe that women in perimenopause who experience migraines with PMS are helped by wearing an estrogen patch or using estrogen cream just before their periods. However, IC patients' reactions to estrogen are individual. Because estrogen increases mast cell secretion of histamines, some IC patients experience a flare-up of symptoms with estrogen. Others find estrogen helpful. *For more information refer to Chapter Eight.*

Migraine patients with IC may need to avoid over-the-counter drugs. Nonsteroidal anti-inflammatory drugs (NSAID's) increase histamine release, and Excedrin and Vanquish contain caffeine. Certain coatings and buffers can also irritate the IC patient's bladder. Prevention of migraine headaches includes following a diet for IC patients, especially the avoidance of foods that contain monosodium glutamate, hot breads, hot raised coffee cakes, hot donuts (cold breads, cakes, and donuts are better), and processed meats. Other triggers for migraines may include fatigue, stress, bright lights, noise, missing meals, hormonal changes, birth control pills, progesterone, and certain fumes from perfume, paint, pesticides, and other toxic products. *Refer to Chapter Six for more information.*

Anti-Inflammatories

Anti-inflammatory medications are sometimes used to treat IC; but often over-the-counter and prescription anti-inflammatory oral medications, intended for the treatment of other conditions, may cause burning in the bladder and stomach upset. Reactions are very individual, but IC patients may want to avoid over-the-counter NSAID's that contain caffeine and other irritating ingredients. *See Treating Migraine Headaches.* Networking and connecting with other IC patients with similar symptoms can be helpful.

Diet Medications and Stimulants

Dieting to lose weight should be combined with exercise and good nutrition, but may not always be appropriate for IC patients. Often IC patients must take prescribed medications which cause a weight increase that is hard to lose. Nevertheless, IC patients should not skip meals or consider taking a diet medication. Diet medications will not only set off IC pain, but will also affect patients who are chemically sensitive. Toxins are stored in fat cells and are mobilized when dieting.

IC patients should try sensible dieting combined with exercise and physician supervision.

Pain Medications

Relieving any type of pain seems to be a challenge for IC patients. Pain medications can contain caffeine and other ingredients which irritate the bladder and stomach. Muscle relaxants prescribed to relieve other muscles in the body (other than the smooth muscle of the bladder) may cause bladder pain and make it difficult for IC patients to fully urinate. Because many medications can adversely affect neurotransmitter levels and bodily functions in IC patients, pain prevention should be used instead as much as possible. *See Coping with General Conditions, Routine Exams and Procedures without the Drugs and Fillers that Might Trigger IC Pain in this chapter.*

Blood Pressure Medications
Medications that treat high blood pressure can trigger IC symptoms. Older medications such as hydralazine seem to be bladder-safe for some patients. The drug Zestril, which is a newer medication, also may be tolerable, but it can cause coughing in some people. Of course, using prevention with diet and exercise, and following a doctor's advice are always recommended.

Chronic Conditions
When IC patients need medication for another chronic condition, they may need to experiment. However, because so many patients have similar overlapping conditions it may be possible to avoid "trial by error." Two fairly common conditions that appear to be treated with IC management are pernicious anemia (B-12 deficiency) and hypothyroidism (low thyroid). Although B-12 deficiency can now be treated with a new prescription oral medication or nasal spray, IC patients may do best with the old-fashioned injections. Unfortunately, even patients diagnosed with pernicious anemia often have to fight for insurance coverage of their injections. Patients with borderline deficiency may also have to convince their doctors to get monthly injections.

IC patients with low thyroid often do best with prescription natural thyroid although different dosages may vary in filler content. The newer and more prescribed brands of synthetic thyroid can trigger bladder symptoms and anxiety in some IC patients. There are arguments pro and con for natural thyroid and a doctor will most probably prefer to prescribe a synthetic make of thyroid. Some IC patients may have to build their thyroid levels slowly. Patients who must cut back on their dosage should also do so slowly.

RESOURCES

New England Compounding Center
(a formulating pharmacy)
1-800-994-NECC (6322)
(508) 820-0606

Dr. Ann McCampbell
(505) 466-3622
www.drannmcc@aol.com

The Vermont Country Store
(802) 362-8440
www.vermontcountrystore.com

Isabella
1-800-777-5205

Chapter 6

UNDERSTANDING CHEMICAL SENSITIVITIES AND ENVIRONMENTAL ILLNESS

Chemicals and toxins are all around us and can have an impact on people with a dysfunctional immune system. Chemicals can also be responsible for a dysfunctional immune system. A number of interstitial cystitis patients experience sensitivity to fragrances and scented products, and occasionally experience bladder symptoms when they are exposed to gasoline fumes, paints and certain chemicals. Some IC patients believe that they suffered with sensitivity before they had IC. Patients with mitral valve prolapse (MVP) and hypothyroidism appear to be more sensitive to chemicals, and recent research has shown a connection between chemical sensitivity and severe fibromyalgia (FMS).

When the presence of antipolymer antibodies (APA) was found in the blood of silicone breast implant patients who suffered with severe FMS symptoms, a group of researchers decided to test the blood of FMS patients who did not have implants. The same antibodies were found in many FMS patients who suffer with severe symptoms. The researchers also learned that breast implant patients who do not experience FMS symptoms do not have the genetic factor which makes other patients chemically sensitive to silicone. APA findings have been mentioned in *The Lancet*, February 1997, volume 349, and in the *Fibromyalgia Wellness Letter* issued by the Arthritis Foundation, April 1999, volume 2. Chemical exposure may now be studied as one possible cause of FMS. *For information on APA testing see Resources in the back of this chapter.*

This chapter will cover the chemical related illness called multiple chemical sensitivity (MCS). Although having IC does not mean that one is, or will become chemically sensitive, this chapter covers a spectrum of sensitivities and makes suggestions in order to try to meet the needs of a varied audience. Also, the following chapter is not limited strictly to the MCS patient, but is instead geared to bring attention to the various environmental factors that may have an impact on some IC patients. Neither is the information in this chapter intended as medical advice nor is it an endorsement of products and services. Many facts and suggestions come from hand-outs shared at support groups, and great effort has been made to give credit, however, in some cases proper credit might have been inadvertently omitted.

What is Multiple Chemical Sensitivity (MCS)?
MCS is defined as a preventable, chronic condition which is marked by a greatly increased sensitivity to multiple chemicals and other irritating substances. For people with MCS, reactions to low levels of common chemicals can be serious, and sometimes life threatening.

What Causes MCS?
MCS may be caused by repeated low-level exposures to chemicals or an acute, high-level exposure to one chemical substance. After such exposure a person may become "sensitized" (develop a sensitivity), or suffer acute reactions to an array of odors and substances. MCS becomes chronic when sensitivity increases.

What are the Symptoms of MCS?
The body is exposed to toxins and allergens through substances that are inhaled, touched, eaten, applied in, or on the body. The most common symptoms of MCS are experienced in the sinuses, respiratory system, and central nervous system.

Symptoms include:

- headaches, including migraines
- hacking coughs
- bronchitis
- dizziness
- tremors
- swelling of the lips, tongue, and eyes
- conjunctivitis
- dermatitis
- fatigue
- cardiac symptoms, such as palpitations and irregular heart beats
- muscle and joint pain
- numbness
- flu-like symptoms and colds
- low grade fever
- depression

Reactions can cause:

- genitourinary problems
- hyper-reactive behavior
- short term memory loss
- hyperactivity in children
- learning disabilities in children

The neurotoxic effects of chemicals can impair functioning. Exposure to certain chemicals, pesticides, and industrial chemicals can lead to liver damage, cancer (including bladder cancer), and damage to the central nervous system. Certain pesticides and detergents contain estrogen-like substances. These substances mimic the effects of estrogen and contribute to an excess of estrogen and an imbalance of hormones in the body.

More information on the symptoms of MCS are available through the research of Grace Ziem, MD, DrPH. *See Resources.*

How is MCS Treated?

Because MCS is best treated with avoidance, it's necessary to read as much as possible in order to make needed lifestyle changes. There are many books that address this illness. Support groups are also helpful and usually have current information. *To find a local support group contact the Human Ecology Action League (HEAL) listed in Resources.*

Environmental consultants, who are knowledgeable about chemical sensitivity, are often necessary when remodeling, building or trying to identify sources of problems in the home and workspace. *To find a consultant contact other MCS patients, environmental or occupational physicians, environmental health departments at local universities or refer to Resources.* In some cities environmental consultants are listed in the yellow pages.

Doctors who specialize in environmental illness are referred to as "environmental physicians" or "occupational physicians." Many of these specialists treat patients with overactive immune dysfunction and degenerative diseases such as systemic lupus, arthritis, and chronic fatigue syndrome (CFS). These physicians are familiar with the limitations of various illnesses, and should respect the IC patient's particularly sensitive needs.

Patients with MCS who are physically able are sometimes advised to exercise and create a sweat in order to mobilize and excrete the toxins stored in the body's fat. A sauna, especially after exercise, to further encourage the release of toxins may also be recommended. This prescription might not be good advice for most IC patients, especially those on dehydrating medications.

Treatments that chelate (attach to a toxin to draw it out of the body) toxins in order to cleanse the body can be very harmful if not done slowly under close supervision. Such treatments should probably be avoided by IC patients because the toxins have to pass through the bladder. IC patients may also have problems with MCS testing and techniques such as Enzyme Potentiated Desensitization (EPD). This technique desensitizes patients to their allergies with immunotherapy, using small doses of allergens. A strict regime and special diet must be followed. EPD may not be advisable for IC patients.

The IC patient's treatment for MCS should be the least intrusive method, which is the avoidance of irritating chemicals. All exercise should be pursued in a clean air environment, because air intake, both good and bad, is increased with exercise. If swimming is a choice, but chlorine is an irritant, find a pool treated by non-chlorinated methods. Local pool companies usually have information on alternative disinfectants; however, some alternatives (such as bromine) can also be irritating. For more information contact the American Environmental Health Foundation, Inc. (AEHF). *Refer to Resources in this chapter as well as Resources in Chapter Three.*

Patients with MCS and IC should avoid any form of fasting. Fasting and regular dieting release toxins because they are stored in the body's fat. If patients must diet for weight loss, it should be a slow process combined with gentle exercise and supervised by their doctors.

Can a Traditional Allergist Help a Patient with MCS?

Most traditional allergists specialize in patients who suffer with traditional allergies and test positive for allergies. Patients who suffer with environmental illness are *sensitive* but not necessarily *allergic*. Even though many MCS patients react to molds and pollens after they become chemically sensitive, they may not test positive for allergies with standard allergy testing.

Traditional allergists may believe that the symptoms of MCS are in a patient's head, or not of an *organic* cause. This idea is sometimes further supported by a patient's behavioral reaction to chemicals and irritants. Reactions to chemicals and irritants can be quite severe, eccentric and very misunderstood. The MCS patient may appear to healthcare professionals as a victim of trauma or abuse. Like IC, MCS is an illness which often requires strong life control, and the need to act quickly and urgently when symptoms are triggered. Also like IC, there is not much known about the illness.

TAKING CONTROL OF YOUR ENVIRONMENT

If you believe that you experience MCS, or would like to improve your environment begin by replacing personal care products that you feel may be irritating. Be sure to read labels carefully before trying new products and remember that no one product or process is assumed safe for everyone with chemical sensitivity.

Personal Care Products

Personal care products are used on, or in your body. They include lotions, cosmetics, nail polish and remover, shampoos and conditioners, gels and hair sprays, perfumes and after shaves, deodorants and soaps, toothpaste and mouthwash. Most scented products today are petrochemical neurotoxins. Ninety-five percent of the chemicals in fragrances are synthetic compounds derived from petroleum. The contents of these fragrances have been found to be capable of causing cancer, birth defects, central nervous system disorders, and allergic reactions. These findings are not new. They were reported in 1986 by the Committee on Science and Technology, U.S. House of Representatives. The EPA is finding more techniques to evaluate the chemicals being used as new products are continually being manufactured. So far only a few chemicals used in fragrances have undergone testing for their carcinogenic effects.

It takes time and money to replace irritating products with suitable ones. Even if your search begins in a health food store, you will probably have to sift through highly scented products and read labels if you wish to avoid silicone compounds. Most cosmetics, shampoos and hair products contain silicone additives. These additives may be listed as dimethicone, simethicone and cyclomethicone. As mentioned earlier, silicone may be harmful to some people. Adverse reactions can cause FMS symptoms, including skin rashes. Many of the less expensive, old fashioned cosmetics and creams do not contain silicone. Companies specializing in natural products sometimes also offer silicone-free products. The company Hope Aesthetics carries two such skin care products that are also not heavily scented, "Gentle Lotion Cleanser" and "Angel's Kiss Cream." The Body Shop, Origins and Clinique also carry some cosmetics, skin care products and shampoos without silicone compounds. Origins and Clinique can be found at department stores. *See Resources to contact Hope Aesthetics and The Body Shop.* Be sure to double check every product.

The comfort of each individual varies and naturally will dictate what should or should not be used. However, it's important to be aware that products labeled *hypoallergenic* do not necessarily protect a person with MCS, and products labeled *unscented* may still contain chemicals and masking fragrances.

Almost any product can affect you if you are sensitive, so it's very important to be conservative when you are trying something new. Always test your body with a small amount at first. You need to be cautious when applying lotions to the buttocks and inner thigh area, and keep in mind that oils and lotions can travel. It is also important to avoid shampooing with strong fragrances or medicated shampoos in the shower. If you are bladder-sensitive, it may be safer to shampoo in the sink to avoid possible contact with the urethra. Bath oils, herbs and bubble bath can irritate the urethra and trigger IC symptoms too. In place of these try adding baking soda or a little sea salt to your bath water. A filtered shower head may be helpful to reduce the amount of chlorine in shower water. Systems to treat the whole home water supply are available. For information on water filters, call the American Environmental Health Foundation, Inc. (AEHF) or National Ecological and Environmental Delivery Systems (N.E.E.D.S). *Refer to Resources.*

Sensitivities are highly individual. When making modifications and replacing products begin with the products you use the most. Be sure to read all new product labels, ingredients and ask questions about everything. Always use your instincts. If you feel the slightest bit uncomfortable with a product, don't use it.

New Clothing

New clothing usually contains strong dyes, dry cleaning solution, masking fragrances, and sometimes fire retardant. Imported clothing may be treated with pesticides. Pure wool may be mothproofed. Even clothing and materials labeled natural or organic aren't always safe.

If you buy a piece of clothing that has a distinct odor or is chemically irritating, you may want to try the following cleaning recipe taken from a support group handout or refer to the book *Less Toxic Living. See Resources.*

- Soak clothing in a bucket of cold water with about ½ cup of powdered milk (do not put powdered milk in the washing machine) for no more than 24 hours.
- Next wash with a tolerated soap.
- Soak clothing for another 24 hours in cold water with ½ cup each of baking soda and white vinegar.
- Rewash in a tolerated soap, and dry.

Wools and silks (not always the linings in clothes) can usually be hand washed in cold water with baking soda or a tolerated soap, however gloves may be necessary. Hang clothes to dry instead of using dryer heat. Heat releases chemicals.

Chemical release also occurs while ironing treated fabrics, so it's necessary to use proper ventilation.

Synthetic clothing can cause itching and irritation. MCS patients should avoid clothing and sheets containing polyester or permanent-press because they may also contain formaldehyde. Dry cleaning is an obvious irritant, but now there are cleaners who use the safer alternative *wet cleaning* which eliminates solvents. Dry cleaners that place *We Care* signs in their windows to show they are taking ecological steps to reduce waste and promote recycling may also offer *wet cleaning*. Sensitive people often wear washable clothing to avoid dry cleaning.

CLEANING UP YOUR HOME ENVIRONMENT

Indoor Air Quality

Your home is important. The better you take care of your needs at home the better you can take care of your life and the people in it.

Many products sold to relieve allergies in the home are intended for people with traditional allergies and not intended for people with chemical sensitivity. Plastic and vinyl covers used to prevent dust mites can make those who are chemically sensitive ill. Instead, a barrier cloth can be used to cover furniture. Sheets and bedding can be washed in hot water to control dust mites and their fecal matter. Organic mattresses, bedding and clothing may be ordered through the Janice Corporation. *See Resources.* Other plastics that emit an odor, such as new shower curtains, shelf paper, etc., may be aired out to decrease the time taken for gases to be released or offgased. However, some new products never stop releasing irritating fumes.

Cleaning Products

Replacing your cleaning products can make life more comfortable instantly. Keeping the environment and air quality clean and free of toxic fumes, mold, mildew, and dust is vital to your health if you are sensitive. Begin changing your cleaning products by replacing chlorine bleach and products containing bleach. Stop using ammonia, commercial floor and furniture polishes, oven cleaners, waxes and strippers. Avoid aerosols and room deodorizers. Avoid all pine scented cleaners and disinfectants.

Hydrogen peroxide can be used in place of bleach. Just substitute ½ of the amount of bleach used with peroxide. There are also some new bleach alternatives that are catching on. Seventh Generation offers a good non-chlorine bleach. *See Resources*. Baking soda is a natural cleaning replacement and can be mixed with water or vinegar for cleaning sink stains and clearing slow drains. Washing soda is another natural cleaner that is useful, and the original Bon Ami is a wonderful bath and kitchen cleaner found at the grocery or health food store. The Bon Ami cleaner and bar are better tolerated than the cleanser. Many new products for cleaning the home are available at health food stores and through catalogs, such as Harmony, The Vermont Country Store, Priorities, and Home Trends. Alternative safe ways of cleaning can be found in the book, "Less Toxic Living." *See Resources*. Remember, it's best to limit the amount of different products you use in your home. Less is considered best.

While cleaning and especially vacuuming, wear a mask to filter out the inhalants of common allergies, such as dust and mold. If vacuuming is always a problem, try using special vacuum cleaner bags that capture allergenic particles or buy a vacuum cleaner with a built-in HEPA filter system. HEPA stands for high-efficiency particulate air filtration. These vacuums are now offered in some commercial stores or through specialty catalogs such as N.E.E.D.S. *See Resources*. Always let a company know that you are chemically sensitive.

Masks and Respirators

Masks and respirators are designed for different purposes. Some masks are helpful to those with dry sinuses, because they retain moisture from the mouth. Some are made to block pollen, mold and dust, but aren't intended to block toxic fumes. These masks may instead trap odors and fumes. Special masks with charcoal inserts should be used to block chemical fumes.

Like everything else, masks may be made of irritating synthetic material. Researching different masks and respirators for your individual needs is necessary. Companies such as N.E.E.D.S or AEHF offer consultation to their customers.

Pesticides

It is very important to avoid exposure to toxic pest control in your environment. Replace insecticide sprays, no-pest strips, moth balls, crystals, and mothproofed paper. They are very toxic. Natural insect repellents such as cedar wood and chips can also irritate those with chemical sensitivity. Replace pest control with alternative products. Minor problems can occasionally be solved with the laundry booster Borax (found in the detergent section in the grocery). Borax sprinkled in cracks and crevices can help to ward off silverfish and eliminate ants when mixed with sugar (keep away from children and pets). Some patients may be sensitive to Borax.

If pesticides are used in your environment, leave until you feel entirely comfortable and experience no side effects upon returning. Chemicals can linger in environments. When buying an older home inquire if it has been treated with the pesticide called Chlordane. This toxic pesticide can last for decades.

In the garden try to fight pests and diseases with garlic sprays and (if tolerated) safe insecticide soaps found in nurseries and at Wal-Mart. Avoid mulch that contains fungicides. Even if you avoid using chemicals in the garden, you may be affected by a nearby golf course or park. To avoid the toxic effects of these areas find out if and when they are sprayed for insects and how the grass is maintained. Stay away at these times.

Foods Treated with Pesticides
The effects from foods treated with pesticides may not be as obvious to those with chemical sensitivity, because symptoms can be delayed. Eating foods that have been grown organically is ideal, however, it's still important for many patients to check if they have been treated with sulfur. It's also important to be aware that farm grown vegetables sold at stands close to busy roadways are exposed to carbon monoxide. It's better to find a natural indoor market that labels ingredients and can answer questions about products. When growing vegetables check the soil for lead content before planting.

For more information on the health effects of pesticides refer to the National Pesticide Telecommunications Network and regional foundations listed in Resources. For chemical-free pest control refer to companies listed under Information, Consultation, Products and Supplies, and Catalogs in Resources.

Canned Goods
Silicone is used in the cleaning process of commercial canned cooked vegetables. Although the vegetables are rinsed off after cleaning, some researchers are studying to see if there is harmful residue left on the vegetables. Soda and beer in cans are also exposed to silicone. These facts may make eating fresh vegetables and drinking from glass bottles a priority for some patients.

Ventilation and Good Air Quality
Airtight homes are not good for anyone. Proper ventilation is necessary to clear the air of chemicals and control the climate. Although it's important to use proper ventilation at all times,

opening windows to outdoor air can often be worse or just not sufficient to clean inside air. People who need to remove organic substances such as mold, dust and pet dander can use a freestanding HEPA filter to clean the air of particulates (some MCS patients do not do well with HEPA filters). Specialized air filters with activated carbon are available to those who need to remove fumes and odors (toxic pollutants). Patients with impaired immune systems should avoid ozone machines for cleaning the air. For specifics about HEPA, specialized air filter systems and different charcoal filters, call N.E.E.D.S. *See Resources.*

Another way to clean environmental air is with an electrostatic filter placed on the central air return. Electrostatic filters can remove small particles of airborne irritants such as mold, bacteria and animal dander, as well as keep indoor air clean during heavy traffic or pollen season when windows are usually shut. It's necessary to clean an electrostatic filter at least every two weeks. This is especially needed in damp climates in order to keep the air flow free and strong enough to reduce moisture.

Your environment is not always easy to control. According to *The Inside Story, A Guide to Indoor Air Quality* (United States Environmental Protection Agency, September 1993), carbon monoxide and other fumes can travel though walls, pipes, floors, cracks, and under doors. Attached garages can allow carbon monoxide to travel into the home even when garage doors are open.

Car exhaust should be kept away from your home and open windows. Venting systems should be checked regularly and furnace filters should be kept clean. Flue gases should also be checked, as well as venting systems and connections. Check oil burners that smell oily, and check all gas burners, ovens and appliances. Keep outside grills away from your house, and gas water heaters housed separately. Avoid gas ovens and appliances. Check them often if you use them. Keep fireplaces clean and open, or close off the chimney and fireplace if they are irritating. Be sure that your clothes dryer vent is clean, clear and vented outside. Consult a mechanical engineer if ventilation problems arise.*

It's necessary for the MCS patient to use good ventilation in the kitchen, because smoke from frying and baking can affect breathing. It's important to keep the oven clean and free of grease. Cooking with organic foods can also help, because chemicals in foods are actually released during the heating process. Avoid using plastic wrap, plastic containers or commercial paper towels in the microwave. Instead use china and microwave safe glass as much as possible.

Contact MCS Referral and Resources for treatment and prevention of low-level carbon monoxide exposure. See Resources.

Eliminating the Items that Expose You to Chemicals in Your Environment

Even with good ventilation, if you have MCS it is necessary to eliminate furniture which contains formaldehyde. It is best to replace or buy solid wood or metal furniture instead. The following furniture contains formaldehyde:

- Furniture made from particleboard
- Furniture made from plywood (unless the plywood has been made without formaldehyde)
- Medium-density fiberboard

Carpeting can also be a big source of formaldehyde and other irritating chemicals. If you can tolerate some carpeting use all cotton or untreated wool, such as Persian or Chinese. Always double check treatments and avoid carpets with rubber backings. Refer to N.E.E.D.S for carpet cleaning in order to avoid chemicals, or just use plain steam to clean carpets. If wall to wall carpeting has been water damaged, it must be replaced.

Other environmental hazards include:

- Mattresses treated with fire retardant, pesticides or fungicides
- Furniture treated with stain guard. Order new upholstered furniture without stain guard. Ask the company to remove the plastic covering and store your new piece of furniture away from chemicals for a couple of weeks until it airs out.
- Treated leather furniture
- Rubber foam cushions

It's very important to avoid fumes and odors while you are sleeping. Become aware of the smaller items and products that have an effect on you.

These items may include:

- Newsprint
- Strong inks
- Glues and tapes

Replace duct tape with aluminum tape or stainless steel adhesive tape. Use white glue like Elmer's Glue or yellow woodworking glue. Be sure to store all chemicals, including paint, in a separate, well ventilated space.

Climate Control
Controlling the humidity in your environment is essential to fight health problems. In the winter months sinuses can become dry and irritated which can result in increased susceptibility to illness.

Steam radiators are preferable to dry forced air which can be very irritating to the sinuses. Most people benefit from the use of a humidifier in the winter months, however, it's necessary to keep humidifiers away from carpeting so it does not become wet. Humidifiers can be placed on tables if necessary. They should be cleaned often with a little vinegar and water. Do not let the humidity in your home get higher than 50%, if possible. Purchase a humidity gauge from a company such as Priorities. *See Resources.*

When the humidity gets too high other problems arise. In the summer months an air conditioner (which is a dehumidifier) and/or a free standing dehumidifier can help to cut down humidity. Filters and ducts must stay clean and free of mold and mildew. Clean your air return filters every couple of weeks. Have your air ducts cleaned at least every ten years, and perhaps more often in damper climates. Avoid using fungicides and harsh chemicals. Look for non-toxic solutions to remove and prevent mildew.

Ceiling fans and other methods of reducing stagnant air such as those mentioned above are helpful, but when air passes over mold, mildew or a dusty area it creates problems. Keep your environment (including vents and fans) clean and properly ventilated. Leave when and if bleaches or other strong cleaning agents are used, and do not return until the fumes have vanished.

Shared Living

MCS patients who live in apartments or condos often must make modifications. Those who live with shared venting may have to cover their vents with aluminum or Denny Foil to keep occasional strong fumes out. When closing off recirculated air, it's often necessary to use a portable heater or window air conditioner. People with MCS need apartment or condo management that is considerate and practices the laws that protect residents under the Fair Housing Act. Residents who are qualified as handicapped can request reasonable accommodations such as being notified before any new work, painting or pest control is started.

Everyone should automatically be notified before new work begins no matter who they are, but most residents in a shared building are not sensitive to the individual resident's needs. However, those with environmental awareness in some progressive cities are promoting environmental-friendly living for individuals in need. No matter, every person should be aware that well-meaning healthy people in charge of projects can innocently replace acceptable products without understanding the consequences to a sensitive person.

THE WORK SPACE

Work performance can be hindered when chemically sensitive people are exposed to chemicals in the workplace.

Modifications for control include:

- Moving your desk away from copy machines and printers
- Avoiding felt-tip pens and using mechanical pencils if you are sensitive to wood bound pencils
- Avoiding instant glues
- Limiting exposure to plastics such as some electrical and electronic equipment with heated surfaces (Chemical residues volatilize with heating.)
- Taking breaks while using such equipment
- Buying a small special air filter for the workspace

There is legal protection for the chemically handicapped at work. Under the Americans with Disabilities (ADA), if an employee has a disability that might interfere with job performance, the employer must assess whether it is possible to "reasonably accommodate" the individual on the job. There may be legal recourse if chemicals are a problem in your workplace and no one will listen.

TRAVEL

Travel is already difficult for most IC patients. When one is also chemically sensitive the following suggestions can be helpful.

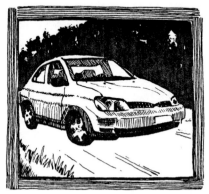

Car Travel

Shut the windows and fresh air vent while driving in heavy traffic or during pollen season. Use the recirculate vent instead. Be aware of sensitivities to the heater, fan, or defroster (the defroster uses outside air). Patients who are sensitive might be more comfortable using the air conditioner. The air conditioner can be set to the warmest temperature when necessary. Sensitive people may also want to start their cars with the air shut off to avoid fumes and/or a pollen shower.

Another way to improve the air quality in your car is with a small specialized charcoal filter air cleaner. Be careful not to use an ozone machine. You do not want to breathe ozone while you are driving, because it may make you lightheaded and confused.

Plane Travel

Sometimes even entering an airport can be offensive. The strong fumes that accompany air travel can make one nauseated, lightheaded, and create breathing problems. Inside a plane there is increased exposure to fumes because one is in a small space that has an artificial source of oxygen. Some people are beginning to wear special, small fresh air machines around their necks. Although these necklaces can provide temporary relief and many people like to use them, they can contain a small amount of ozone. Ozone may not be good for patients with MCS. *For information call the AEHF in Resources.* For general information on plane travel send for the book, *Jet Smarter,* by Diana Fairechild. *See Resources under Travel.*

Hotel Stays

You can request a non-smoking room, and ask for no air fresheners, scents (place all soaps in a drawer), sprays, ozone machines, newly painted or renovated rooms when you make hotel reservations. You can request your reserved room to be aired in advance, if the windows open. You can also bring extra pillow cases and your own pillow to avoid strong bleach or scented fumes in bedding.

Although hotel stays can be challenging, you may be more comfortable staying in a hotel than in a friend's home. It's usually easier to ask for what you need in a hotel. *For more information, see Hotel Stays in Resources.*

BUILDING OR REMODELING A TOXIC-FREE HOME

When building or remodeling, it is essential for people with chemical sensitivity to check all building materials carefully before using. Particleboard, plywood (some of the newer plywood may be made without formaldehyde), and medium-density fiberboard are big sources of formaldehyde. To avoid formaldehyde, ask stores or companies for a copy of the MSDS for product contents. Replace plywood with outdoor plywood unless indoor plywood has no formaldehyde. Use solid wood, steel, or enamel cabinets. Avoid wood veneers and vinyl coated cabinets. Counters should be made of tile, granite or solid wood.

Use ceramic tiles on floors instead of vinyl. Use hard wood floors instead of wall to wall carpeting. Seal wood only with a water based urethane, paint or clear resin. Although clear varnishes are better than stains, they still need time to off-gas toxic fumes.

Building products need to be well researched for your individual needs. Specialized plant and milk based paints are now available for the chemically sensitive, however, latex paints that are considered low-odor can still have strong fumes. Some patients must avoid latex paints and all IC patients should avoid oil based paints. Silicones can be a problem and the fumes can take time to dissipate, or off-gas. Drywall compound may be okay, but patients may not be able to tolerate wallpaper made of vinyl, and/or find that plain wallpaper causes problems if the glue under the paper mildews. It's usually wise to avoid using wallpaper in damp areas and rooms without windows. When fiberglass insulation is used, it's important that it is contained and wrapped tightly to keep formaldehyde from emitting toxic gases.

Ideally, your new home or addition should be free of gas appliances and heaters. Solar and electric heat, air conditioning and appliances are healthier. Most homes can be converted from gas to electricity. If you build a new home or addition be sure that it is well ventilated with outdoor air supplies to the kitchen, bath and laundry area. Living well is necessary and often difficult. Recognizing your needs is the first step and taking action is the second and most important step. *Refer to A Toxic-Free Home in Resources.*

RESOURCES

APA Information and Testing

Autoimmune Technologies
144 Elks Place
Suite 1402
New Orleans, LA 70112
(504) 529-9944
www.autoimmune.com

National MCS Organizations

HEAL (Human Ecology Action League)
P.O. Box 29629
Atlanta, GA 30359-0629
(404) 248-1898
E-Mail Address: HEALNatnl@aol.com
(contact *HEAL* for support chapters and newsletters)

NCEHS (National Center for Environmental Health Strategies)
1100 Rural Avenue
Voohees, NJ 08043
(609) 429-5358
E-Mail Address: WJRD37A@prodigy.com
(newsletters)

CIIN (Chemical Injury Information Network)
P.O. Box 301
White Sulfur Springs, MT 59645
(406) 547-2255

Books

Less Toxic Living
Carolyn P. Gorman
To order: (214) 368-4132 or 1-800-634-1380

Chemical Exposures, Low Levels and High Stakes
Nicholas Ashford and Claudia Miller (second edition, John Wiley & Son, Inc.) 1998

Staying Well in a Toxic World
Lynn Lawson (The Noble Press, Inc. Chicago) 1993

Information, Consultation, Products, and Supplies

Always indicate that you are ordering for a MCS person and would like your products and wrappings fragrance-free. Inquire about return policies.

American Environmental Health Foundation, Inc. (AEHF)
1-800-428-2343
(supplies and products)

MCS Referral and Resources (Multiple Chemical Sensitivity Referral & Resources)
(410) 362-6400
www.mcsrr.org

Dr. Grace Ziem
(301) 241-4346

Environmental Education and Health Services, Inc.
(512) 288-2369
(telephone and onsite consultation)

N.E.E.D.S (National Ecological and Environmental Delivery Systems)
1-800-634-1380
needs@needs.com
(products and catalogs)

Harmony
1-800-869-3446
(products and catalogs)

Janice Corporation
1-800-526-4237
(products, including Seventh Generation, and catalogs)

Nigra Enterprises
(818) 889-6877
(products and consultation)

Catalogs and Products not Specifically for MCS

Hope Aesthetics Cosmeceutical, Inc.
1-800-266-4799

The Body Shop
1-800-263-9746

Priorties
1-800-553-5398

The Vermont Country Store
(802) 362-8440
www.vermontcountrystore.com

Alsto's Handy Helpers
1-800-447-0048

Improvements
1-800-642-2112

Home Trends
1-800-810-2340

Pesticide Information

National Pesticide Telecommunications Network
1-800-858-PEST (7378)
(effects of pesticides)

New York Coalition For Alternative To Pesticides (NYCAP)
(518) 426-8246

National Coalition Against The Misuse Of Pesticides (NCAMP)
(202) 543-5450

Travel

Jet Smarter
Diana Fairechild
Magellan's
1-800-962-4943
(travel supplies)

Evergreen Rooms
1-800-929-2626

Hospitality Plus
(This travel guide can be ordered from *HEAL*. *See National MCS Organizations.*)

A Toxic-Free Home

Healthy House Institute
(812) 332-5073

Green Resource Center
(510) 845-0472

Please note that "Angels Kiss Cream", mentioned on Page 101, contains dimethicone. Products in this book may change periodically. Read all labels carefully and request ingredients when ordering over the phone or online.

Chapter 7
IDENTIFYING, CONTROLLING AND AVOIDING IC SYMPTOMS WITH SELF-HELP

Pain is Motivation to Change
Almost every IC patient will agree that they would rather go through anything else but the pain of a bad IC flare-up. While it's normal for new patients to first wonder why and how they got interstitial cystitis, as they become engrossed in the process of finding a successful treatment their focus usually changes to recognizing and identifying the particular factors and culprits that set off their IC symptoms.

With the right knowledge, IC patients quickly learn to understand their painful flare-ups and even sometimes predict their durations as they become more familiar with this disease. Unfortunately, there are still many helpful suggestions that patients may overlook when they do not need help for a particular symptom. The following tips are intended to give more control to individuals who learn to turn to themselves for relief and prevention.

COPING WITH URGENCY AND FREQUENCY

Two self-help techniques for IC patients who experience urgency and frequency are bladder training and double voiding.

Bladder Training
Bladder training actually can be effective for patients who experience frequency and poor emptying caused by muscle

damage. Damage occurs from frequently voiding a bladder that isn't able to hold a small amount of urine without pain, pressure and/or frequency (a normal bladder holds about a pint of urine for a couple of hours). Bladder training helps to strengthen the bladder muscle, improve circulation and increase bladder capacity, all of which may restore a more comfortable voiding pattern. With practice, patients usually experience improvement in several weeks.

Experts advise IC patients to add a few minutes to their intervals between voiding in order to retrain the bladder nerves and muscles, and increase bladder capacity. Obviously this protocol should not be practiced while one is in pain or experiencing the first challenges of IC. And, like other treatments, it may not be right for every patient. Some IC patients find distraction the best tool to use while lengthening interval times.

Everyone with IC has experienced a situation when they have had to hold urine just a little longer than they would like. When this occurs, their urine stream often becomes stronger when they finally void. They also may find they can empty their bladder more fully, and sometimes do not feel the urge to void again as soon. The longer interval has actually helped their bladder to function better.

However, the opposite can happen when patients who suffer with frequency and urgency have had to wait so long that they experience pain. When this happens there may be difficulty beginning a urine stream or fully voiding. In this case the bladder has become distended (this can happen overnight as well) which can be very painful and cause spasms. Bladder training needs to be practiced slowly and comfortably in order to strengthen the urine stream, reduce urgency and help to calm a frequency cycle. Bladder training is best used in conjunction with other medications and treatments for IC.

Double Voiding

Patients who have the urgency to void again right after they urinate usually cannot void fully. Even the smallest amount of urine can be an irritant, add pressure and create the urgent need to empty the bladder again. By taking time after finishing a urine stream to void a second time, most IC patients find they can empty their bladders more fully, and therefore, reduce the pressure that creates the urgency to void again.

If you try double voiding, wait several seconds after you have completed your first void, relax and then without straining, try to void again. Use different methods to encourage a second void, such as deep breathing, visualization, shifting your sitting position, stretching your upper body, or picking up a magazine to shift your mind away from the task. The toilet is also a safe place to try deep breathing into your belly without the worry that you will have to void.

There are two methods that may be used to help empty a stubborn bladder. One is the Credé maneuver which is done by applying pressure to the lower abdomen with hands facing each other and fingers spread, somewhat overlapping. The other method is the Valsalva maneuver which requires bending forward over the thighs to create pressure on the lower abdomen before voiding. The Valsalva method may be more comfortable for IC patients.

Although these methods can work, double voiding without straining is the safest and the healthiest way to empty your bladder. The pressure used in the Credé maneuver and the Valsalva maneuver can force urine back up into the ureters in some people. IC patients who have acid reflux may not be candidates for these maneuvers also. Patients who would like to try these methods should talk to their doctors.

PAINFUL FLARE-UPS

Although patients become acutely attentive to their IC management, they may find that controlling the symptoms of IC is
like playing the children's game, "Mother May I." Symptoms
can get out of control and flare-ups can just happen.

The disease, the bladder pain and the management of IC
are different for each patient. Depending on the individual
some pain may be managed in a few hours or overnight. But
there are times when bladder pain develops into a nasty flare-
up. When this happens the flare-up has all of the individual's
attention, controlling both mind and body.

IC flare-ups may involve pressure, urgency, frequency,
burning, stinging, urethral, bladder, and pelvic floor spasms, as
well as pain in the vagina (or penis and scrotum), perineum,
and/or rectum. Patients may experience referred low back and
leg pain, and a feeling of weakness and shakiness in their torso,
hips, and/or legs. Some patients also describe a pulling sensation in their pelvic floor and an overall experience of feeling
held up in a tension pattern. IC symptoms have been compared
to having a knife turning in the bladder, ground glass in the
bladder, a lit match, an ant pile, a bladder migraine, a relentless
nagging sensation, dryness, soreness, and a throbbing feeling.

Although symptoms vary from patient to patient, everyone affected can agree that when the pain comes, it's like having a dark veil dropped over the spirit. Everything can look and
feel different the minute the pain begins. A patient may feel as
if she or he has been taken from the present surroundings, isolated and shut down. This experience can happen very quickly,
and cause fear and anxiety about the next moment, future re-
sponsibilities, expectations, and duration of the pain.

Pain leads to changes in the central nervous system.
There is a great need to act quickly, and to deal with the present
as a *fight or flight* reaction takes place in the body. Figuring
how and why the pain has happened is normal. A flare-up is a

very big disappointment to the IC patient and often to those around her or him. Feelings of guilt or self-blame can make the reaction to the pain worse. The focus must be on pain relief. Pain is never healthy, even in minimal amounts. Pain is a signal to do something quickly to stop it, and ultimately, to stop doing something that may be causing it.

Treating a Flare-Up

IC patients treat and cope with their flare-ups in different ways. Some patients need to retire and put their feet up when IC symptoms begin to flare. Some drink a lot of water to dilute their urine or wash away the irritant. Some patients quit drinking water to stop urgency and frequency and, some drink baking soda (one teaspoon in a glass of water) or take Tums to neutralize the urine. Other patients take medication immediately or may need a combination of treatments.

The following information details various problem-solving and coping techniques that IC patients use to treat the different degrees and symptoms of a flare-up.

Reclining to Relieve IC
and Associated Muscle Weakness

Feeling weakness and shakiness in your muscles is a signal which tells you that you are overextending yourself. Weakness and shakiness should also be a cue for you to get off your feet and lie down so that you can relieve the tension in your postural muscles. Although your body will be fully supported while you are lying down, you will need additional support for your upper back, neck, head, and arms if you read or watch TV. Using a bed wedge may be helpful. You can usually find these large wedges in stores or catalogs specializing in products for your back. For optimum support when using a bed wedge, place a pillow under your head and another one on your stomach to support a book if you are reading. The angle of the wedge should place your abdominal muscles in slack and allow them to rest. The longer the bed wedge, the better for your body. If your bed wedge puts pressure on your sacrum and tailbone add a small folded towel to make the wedge longer. *Refer to The Vermont Country Store (see Resources in Chapter Two) for different styles of wedges and support pillows.*

When you need to rest flat on the bed try a jack knife position. Turn on your side and bring your legs straight out in front of you. This position will put your abdominal muscles in slack and stretch out your low back, buttocks and hamstring muscles. You can also stretch your hip flexors (which is very important) in this position by bringing one leg straight under your body while leaving the other straight out in front. To increase this stretch, bend your knees. No matter how you relieve a flare-up make sure that you incorporate proper support for your body while you're in a tension pattern.

Cold and Heat Therapy
for Bladder Spasms and Burning

Typically the rule is cold for inflammation and heat for muscle spasms. Cold constricts the blood vessels which reduces the flow of blood to the area and helps to slow the body's response to inflammation. IC patients, however, seem to vary in their preferences. Some women reduce bladder pain and burning by holding a cold pack just above the clitoris for 15 to 20 minutes. Relief is often not felt until the cold pack is lifted away. Patients may prefer to avoid contact with the sensitive genital areas while using cold packs. Wrapping the cold pack with a thick towel can make the pack more comfortable, as well as prevent frostbite.

Other IC patients find relief by placing a cold or hot pack on the perineum area between the anus and vagina (between the anus and base of the penis in men) to relieve bladder pain. Patients who are prone to yeast infections may not be candidates for heat in this area. Some patients prefer to use heat on their low back or abdomen, or use a heated mattress pad to relieve the whole body effect of IC pain. It's important to be cautious because too much heat is not good for inflammation. Moist heat is best for the bladder and pelvic floor. Both hot and cold packs should last the appropriate therapeutic time, about 20 minutes. Either can be replaced again after another 20 or 30 minutes if necessary.

The benefits of hot and cold are not entirely limited to external use. Drinking a hot beverage in the morning can relax the bladder muscle and help to dilute concentrated urine. Eating cold ice cream helps some patients during a flare-up. Of course, hot and cold drinks and food must be bladder-safe for the individual. Experience and preference is unique to each IC patient.

Neutralizing Your Urine to Treat Burning

Taking a teaspoon of baking soda in a glass of water can help to neutralize urine for about eight hours. Taking two Tums also helps to neutralize acidic urine. And, the product Prelief can also be used for acid-reduction. Neutralizing the urine is often used as pain prevention. It's necessary, however, to inform doctors and pharmacists when using these treatments because they may interfere with the effects of prescription drugs. If neutralizing your urine is helpful, your doctor may prescribe a medication such as Tagamet for this treatment. (Tagamet has been known to create bladder pain in some IC patients.) *See Chapter Two for more information.*

Relieving Bladder Spasms with a Bladder Massage

A bladder massage may not sound very comfortable, but it can help to calm uncomfortable spasms. This massage technique is best performed by a partner or a massage therapist. It is very simple. Following the top edge of the pubic bone (the bone in front of the bladder) from one side to the other, make small, circular massage strokes upward toward the belly with two or three fingers. Repeat these strokes as many times as needed and then massage the tight areas on each side of the bone where the legs join. Follow these tight areas down and then upward toward the hips.

The bladder massage can help to relax a contracted bladder as well as the surrounding muscles. This technique works very well in conjunction with medication, or for some patients, alone. Massage work in general can be helpful in breaking a tension pattern.

WHEN FLARE-UPS TURN INTO PAIN CYCLE

Scheduling a Treatment or Appointment

When there is little relief from a flare-up day after day, many IC patients call their urologists to schedule a treatment or ask for a new medication.

It's necessary to have a doctor who offers immediate treatment, especially for the patient who depends on bladder instillations for relief. As any IC patient knows, symptoms are often unpredictable and flare-ups can be a surprise. The ideal doctor will believe you, encourage your IC management and give you positive feedback, as well as relief. The IC patient needs a doctor who can accept the whole picture of her or his illness. Unfortunately, this doesn't always happen.

Many patients with chronic conditions get negative responses from doctors so they learn to edit or hold back information. Chronic pain patients often must seek approval to get help. However, patients with the pain of IC cannot spare a moment to get another person's approval. Insisting on immediate care will not work with many doctors, but if IC patients are too calm their pain may not be recognized or treated. Office visits can end up seeming like a balancing act. Receptionists and doctors who do not understand IC may see patients as extremely emotional. This includes some urologists. Most IC patients can get oral medications from other doctors, such as primary care physicians, if they cannot find the right urologist. Patients not dependent on urologists for treatments may do better by working with other doctors who are available to their needs.

IC patients who depend on bladder instillations to relieve their IC symptoms can learn to instill their own medicines. In many cases, self-catheterization can provide fast relief, as well as a greater sense of control. Sometimes self-catheterization is necessary for IC patients who live too far from their doctors' offices. Patients should talk to their urologists if they feel self-catheterization might be helpful. Medications should never be instilled into the bladder when patients have urinary tract infections.

Contact Another IC Patient

Avoid suffering in silence. It's easy to lose perspective when you are in IC pain. Another IC patient will understand, remind you that you will feel better and often give you helpful suggestions. Being able to communicate your symptoms, and express how they make you feel may help to begin a healing process. Staying in touch with another IC patient while you seek medical help can also be reassuring and empowering. No one else can understand your situation as well as another IC patient.

When Your Pain Cycle Causes
More Stress in Your Life

After a few days of pain a person's whole body takes on a tension pattern. It is very important to try to release this tension, because it can create a vicious cycle that in turn will increase your IC pain. If you are worn-out from IC pain it is vital to eliminate extra stress. Taking time out will make it possible to take strong medications when they would otherwise interfere with typical everyday functions. On a more normal day, work and daily routines may serve as helpful distractions, but taking time out for yourself when you're in a lot of pain is necessary both physically and mentally. It is very important to accept the fact that you will experience down days and will need backup help just for these times.

Get Out of Your Environment

A stubborn pain cycle is a vicious cycle. If you have been house bound and your pain isn't improving, it's sometimes necessary to get out of your environment. Get dressed, put on makeup or whatever you usually do before going out, and then leave the house for a little while. You may benefit from a change of scenery. Because change can help you to feel a shift in your emotions, it can have a positive physical effect in breaking a pain cycle. Getting involved and participating in something a little different can also help.

Fatigue the Pain Pattern

For some patients the only way to beat the pain of IC is to match it, wear it down. The false energy or hyper feeling some IC patients experience with their bladder pain can cause them to pace. When one finds it difficult to sit still, is exhausted from the tension in their body and can not find relief with medication or relaxation techniques, it sometimes works to fatigue the muscles naturally through appropriate movement.

One way to fatigue muscles is by walking at a fast pace (not power walking). Taking a short walk close to home can also help to break a frequency cycle. Patients who are unable to walk because of the impact to their bladders may want to try other forms of movement. Stretching and free-form dancing, a dance video or another form of comfortable exercise done in the home can serve as an alternative. Turn on music. Music is movement and can help to cycle patients out of a pattern. The goal of movement is to fatigue the pain, to tire out the pattern in the muscles, to increase circulation, encourage full breathing, and produce endorphins, which can help to repair the effect IC has on the limbic system.

Recognizing Your Pain Triggers

When you can't pinpoint the cause of an ongoing pain pattern it can be frustrating to try to make sense of it or find a way to stop it. But you can help yourself by reviewing the different culprits reported as pain triggers by IC patients. If you can pinpoint and make yourself aware of your triggers you can hopefully stop, better cope with, and prevent some future flare-ups.

Various Pain Triggers

- Diet changes, including drinking water and ice (Be aware that city tap water changes periodically in chlorine content and is susceptible to chemical spills.)
- Adverse reactions to medications
- Menstrual cycle
- Perimenopause and menopause
- Stress
- Overextending yourself physically or emotionally
- Sexual activity
- Changes in dietary tolerance
- Lack of good sleep
- Urinary tract infection
- Yeast infection
- Dehydration
- Adverse reactions to new therapies
- Adverse reactions to new exercise
- New activities including house and yard work
- Travel
- Adverse reactions to new environments, chemicals, paints, home improvements, pesticides, gasoline, etc.
- Seasonal changes, weather changes
- Poor ergonomics, lack of good support while active or resting

- Tight pants that pull your hips back and under when sitting, or pants that hold your buttocks too close together

ILLNESS BREAKS THE RULES

Dealing with People

Having IC means dealing with more than physical pain. Explaining the effects that IC has on your life may be the second hardest challenge, because of the response you get. People who have not been exposed to chronic illness will most probably have a difficult time understanding your pain, needs and lifestyle.

How well other people understand your IC can also depend on how well you accept and deal with your own illness. There are many different factors that play into your acceptance of IC. These factors can include your background, cultural values and beliefs, the role you play in your family, career demands, self-expectations, age, how you've dealt with illness in the past, reactions of family, friends, employers, co-workers, and of course, your doctors. When these factors interfere with your self-care they are a problem.

IC requires strict coping skills and it's often necessary to remind the people around you that you have to stay on top of your condition. IC is invisible to others, but usually when people spend enough time with you they find that you are more accessible when you are in control of your own needs. Still at first, you may have to ask for a lot, sift through people and their opinions, and take control before you earn the understanding of those affected by your IC. Although there may be those who will feel resentful and controlled by your needs, you must remind yourself that you are not responsible for their reactions. If you do not take good care of yourself, you won't be able to take care of anyone or anything else.

You may be often told you lack confidence when you are fearful of taking long car rides, getting in the car with another driver, going to new restaurants, taking trips, or starting new employment. People with this opinion do not understand the complexity of IC. They do not know how much confidence, willpower and determination living with IC takes. Confidence in yourself is a multifaceted issue. You can be completely secure and assertive in certain situations, but not in other situations in which you do not have access to, or know where a bathroom is within a limited time frame.

In general, IC patients tend to be most confident when they are not rushed and can control their environment in relationship to their bladder needs. When others label an IC patient as "unconfident" or "not trying" they do not understand this complex disease.

It's essential to educate those around you and make them aware of your unique lifestyle management. You may need to set new boundaries and even make new friends. Learn to represent your new life without being negative. If you can accept your illness, limitations and modified lifestyle (this does not mean accepting the pain) you will gain admiration and support from most people.

At times, you may have to depend on people you don't care for, such as skeptical and difficult healthcare professionals, insurance companies and even family members. Because of this dependence it's essential (when at all possible) to avoid other people who do not believe that you are limited by IC. Seeking out supportive people that understand and accept you is necessary because if you don't feel good about yourself when you're with someone, they are NOT GOOD FOR YOU!

Finding Support

Treating your physical symptoms is the first step of self-help. Treating your emotional pain may be the second. Blame is handed out too easily to victims and at times unconditional love from family and friends isn't there. A good support group can really help this situation. Find a group that actively listens to you and a group that works to improve the quality of life for people with IC and other chronic conditions. A good group can offer unconditional support, help you to build a new sense of self-awareness and control, help you to become assertive and inquisitive, and perhaps provide you with some nice new friends. All of this will protect you from the impact of negativity that can exist with IC. If you cannot find a local IC support group start one by placing an ad in your paper or get on the internet.

In addition to support groups, mental health professionals such as social workers or psychologists can also help you deal with your disease. Therapists who work with chronic pain patients have expertise in offering practical lifestyle management strategies which can help both your physical and emotional pain. It is important to find a professional who uses effective counseling, which incorporates dialogue between the therapist and patient.

It is also necessary to understand the difference between a psychologist and a psychiatrist when choosing an appropriate mental health practitioner. A psychiatrist is a medical doctor with additional training in psychology. Be aware that many psychiatrists have an analytic orientation which will not meet your needs if you are looking for a therapist who will actively provide feedback and suggestions. Psychiatrists, however, have expertise with psychotropic medications such as antidepressants and anti-anxiety medications. Consultations with a psychiatrist may help you find the most effective psychotropic medication with the fewest side effects.

Successes Improve the Quality of Life

Successes and accomplishments are necessary to achieve a feeling of involvement and productivity. Without them, life's problems can become overwhelming and depressing. To achieve success you first must know yourself and your limitations. You must accept and understand your unique symptoms to reach your goals realistically. If you learn to manage your time, avoid overextending yourself and seek out safe environments, you can successfully control the daily impact of IC. When you accomplish more, you will feel a sense of satisfaction.

Successes are more easily achieved when you become more cognizant of your body's tension patterns. When you use proper support and stay physically strong, you can accomplish more. Try to incorporate a comfortable home exercise program. Select music and a comfortable exercise mat. Even if you can only exercise one or two days a week, making the effort will improve the quality of your life, release stress, give you renewed energy, and will reward you with a sense of accomplishment. Success leads to commitment.

Self-Expression is Necessary

When life's priorities change with IC, so can your perspective and values. Although the smaller pleasures may take on more meaning for you, you live in an extremely competitive society. You can have a difficult time finding where you fit in, as well as finding your meaning and purpose in our goal oriented world. You may find it necessary to discover new interests and outlets, new forms of escape and ways to express yourself. Because your life has changed so much you may do this quite successfully. Whether it's painting, drawing, studying a new topic, pursuing a new hobby or exercise routine, or helping others in need, self-expression is a necessary component to stress management. Self-expression can minimize the mundane chore of dealing with physical problems, as well as affirm your role in society.

Seek Comfort and Make Life Easier

- Wear comfortable clothes. Buy slacks a size larger to get more room in the crotch. You can take them in elsewhere.

Use scissors and make little downward slits in elastic waist bands to make more room.

- Empty your bladder before meals if you experience frequency and pressure. Eating should not be rushed. You do not need to anticipate a trip to the bathroom.
- Carry a portable urinal in the car, even if it's only for peace of mind.
- Wear a pad or guard under your clothes if you aren't sure about restroom accessibility.
- Carry a medic alert bracelet with "interstitial cystitis" engraved in it, a letter of verification from your doctor or a bathroom pass from the ICA to gain access to a restroom or to the front of a line when needed. (Providing ID passes for IC and other patients for restroom access in businesses and other commercial facilities is in legislation in some states.)
- Ask your doctor to help you get a handicapped parking permit. Because IC is not usually accepted as a handicap you may have better luck requesting a permit for an overlapping condition. For information call your state motor vehicle department.
- Find a drug and grocery store that can deliver when you need help. The extra expense can be a tradeoff or prevention for days missed at work, co-pays for doctor visits and medicines.
- Call your post office about Stamps By Mail or use www.stamps.com. Post office lines can be challenging.
- Find a cleaning person to help with difficult chores at least once a month, if possible. (Some IC patients are able to barter for services.) Often chronic pain patients who must stay at home are expected to do all of the housework!
- If you are seeing a very busy doctor, call ahead of your appointment to see if the doctor is running on time.
- Always ask your doctor to write down what you don't understand.

- Take notes so you don't forget important information from your doctor.
- Contact the ICA for a local support group, for its ICA Update reports, and information on research fund raising.
- Contact the IC Network for its IC Handbook, patient chat room, and for its doctor question and answer corner.
- Read books on IC.
- Read books on coping with chronic illnesses.
- Refer to the Americans with Disabilities Act (ADA) if you experience discrimination for time taken from work for treatments and medical leave, or for being turned away for a position.
- If you can no longer work, apply for Social Security Disability.* You will need one or two very thorough doctors to help you, although you will be required to list all of the doctors who treat your conditions.

Make sure your doctors understand the extent of your disability, including limitations in sitting, standing, walking, lifting, driving, working, and environmental sensitivities. Follow the suggestions for fibromyalgia (FMS) documentation reported in the July 1999 issue of *The Fibromyalgia Network:*

1. Visit your urologist at least three times a year.
2. Make a list (typed, if at all possible) of your current symptoms for each visit. Give one copy to the doctor; keep a copy for your personal records. Also include in that list, any problems you are experiencing that interfere with your day to day functioning such as riding in a car, working, housework, social activities, etc. Go over this list with your doctor and ask that it be included in your medical records.
3. Make this a habit you practice with all of the doctors, counselors and/or therapists you see.
4. Make personal notes or keep a diary.

* *The IC patient should be prepared to be denied benefits the first and maybe the second time. At this point, it is necessary to find a disability lawyer for representation. The lawyer will not require payment but will be entitled to a percentage of disability payments from the time the patient was out of work to the time she or he goes to court. Contact the ICA or IC Network for more information.*

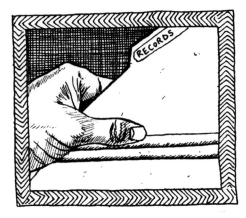

Chapter 8
MANAGING SEX, MENOPAUSE, PREGNANCY AND IC

SEX AND IC

A majority of IC patients experience *dyspareunia* which means painful intercourse. Painful sex is not exclusive to heterosexual intercourse and can be experienced with stimulation and fore-play, insertion, penetration, and/or orgasm. Pain can occur after sex and sometimes sets off a pain cycle.

There are actually three categories regarding the cycle of sexual response. The first phase is the desire phase. Second is the excitement phase and third is the orgasm phase. Although having IC does not necessarily affect sexual function, the asso-ciated pain, as well as certain medications and treatments, can interfere with libido and performance in both sexes. Patients who experience pain with sexual activity often become vigilant and protective, needing to keep a close watch during their sex-ual involvement. Although the pain that occurs with sexual ac-tivity is very real and physical in origin, emotional effects may stem from the fear of pain, the pressure to perform, and a chal-lenged sexual identity.

Pain is a signal to make one aware that something isn't working as it should. Generally, painful sex in IC patients is caused by an irritation in the bladder, but there are many IC pa-tients who have overlapping conditions that add to painful sex. Among these is a common condition called *pelvic floor dysfunc-tion* (PFD), or *vaginismus* which causes the pelvic floor muscles to contract abnormally in response to an irritant. PFD is also associated with and/or contributes to some of the other over-lapping conditions covered in this chapter.

How IC Causes Painful Sex

The reason sexual stimulation and intercourse cause pain in IC patients has to do with several factors such as the obvious one, the proximity of the bladder and the pelvis. During sexual excitement and stimulation, pelvic organs and the surrounding tissue of the genitalia are affected. When their bodies prepare for intercourse with lubrication and an increased blood flow into the genital area, IC patients may begin to experience pain. IC patients seem to have a particular sensitivity to vasoconstriction because of the massive capillary growth and numerous blood vessels in their inflamed bladders. Another reason for pain during the excitement phase is muscle spasm, due to irritated muscles that don't contract and expand as they should in preparation for orgasm. Pain experienced during the excitement phase can interfere with intercourse.

Denise Webster RN, PhD, CS, in her article *Sex and Interstitial Cystitis: Explaining the Pain and Planning Self-Care*, points out Gillespie's theory that muscles spasm or become hyperactive during intercourse because the nerve pathways in the bladder become involved when the irritation is stimulated during intercourse. However, Gillespie also suggests that IC patients may experience a *temporary* relief from IC pain while having an orgasm, because the nerves are inhibited during this time. Whether this happens or not, having an orgasm can often lead to bladder pain after sex. IC patients may have to stay detached in order to prevent orgasm.

Orgasm in women involves contraction of the walls of the outer vagina, uterus, clitoris, urethra and bladder, as well as the sphincter muscle of the rectum. In men muscle contractions involve the ducts connecting the testes, the prostrate and the penis when forcing the semen out.

Normally after orgasm blood is pumped away from the pelvic area, organs relax and return to normal size. However, IC patients can experience prolonged vasoconstriction, and women may have pain and throbbing in the clitoris, bladder, urethra, and behind the vagina. Males with IC can experience pain at the tip of the penis and in the testicles. Other symptoms that occur after orgasm may include frequency, burning, low back, and leg pain. Because of the inflammatory condition in the bladder, orgasm can trigger a flare-up. Some IC patients simply must avoid sexual intercourse. Others find ways to prevent and/or minimize pain.

Medical Diagnosis and Treatment

Although it doesn't take a doctor to tell the IC patient they have a painful condition that causes pelvic floor spasms, there is a pelvic exam to confirm a diagnosis of abnormal contraction of pelvic floor muscles. During the exam the doctor palpates point tenderness or trigger points in the vagina in a woman, or the rectum in a man. The exam includes palpation of the very tight, and usually weak, sensitive muscles in the IC patient called the pubococcygeal muscles, or PC. This exam can be painful and can also trigger referred pain into the bladder, hips, low back, and legs. You may want to tell your doctor that you do not need confirmation of your condition.

Treatment for PFD includes standard treatment for IC and overlapping conditions, prescribed antispasmodic drugs, muscle relaxants, numbing agents during sex to allow more comfort during insertion and penetration, electrical stimulation to stabilize the muscles *(see Standard Treatments in Chapter One)*, and special muscle therapy on the pelvic floor. Specific massage and treatment for PFD are offered by some physical therapists and practitioners in pain clinics. For optimum relief, hands-on work should address the tissue surrounding the ramus, the gluteal attachments, the deep lateral rotator muscles, especially the piriformis, the ischial tuberosities and the hip flexors. Therapists should avoid putting direct pressure on joint areas especially near the sacral nerves. *Refer to physical therapy clin-*

ics, the ICA and the IC Network for information on pelvic floor
massage and therapy.

INTERCOURSE AND PAIN MANAGEMENT

Warming your Muscles Before Intercourse

If you are able to have sexual intercourse but need to avoid the
stimulation of foreplay, you might follow the suggestion of
some doctors and use a warm gel pack (not too hot) on your
pelvic floor for five to ten minutes before intercourse. The
warmth can help to provide an even blood supply and help to
relax the pelvic floor muscles. If planning and waiting for sex
leads to anticipation and anxiety, you might prefer to forego this
step.

Proper Lubrication

Adequate lubrication is necessary to avoid irritation to sensitive
tissues and tight muscles. If you buy over-the-counter lubricants be sure they are water based, although there is no guarantee that all water based lubricants will be bladder-safe. You
might find the lubricant "Slippery Stuff" the least irritating. *See
Resources at the end of this chapter.*

Pure safflower oil is another alternative to commercial
brands of lubrication, however, it's necessary to keep natural
oils fresh and refrigerated. When trying something new always
be sure to use a very small amount and apply as far from the
urethra as possible.

Medications and Numbing Agents

Antispasmodics and other pain medications taken before or after intercourse may help reduce spasms and pain, as well as help
patients to void more fully after intercourse. Before intercourse,
some IC patients use a topical anesthetic such as lidocaine to
numb the genital area. Although numbing agents aid relaxation
and block pain during intercourse, not all IC patients may be

able to tolerate them or they may also need to take medication to relieve burning and spasms afterwards. Topical cortisone which can help reduce swelling after intercourse can be a bladder irritant to IC patients. It's vital to use one medication or product at a time in order to determine what is helpful and what might cause irritation and pain.

Birth Control

Preventive measures can be a challenge for IC patients. Birth control pills contain progestational (progesterone) agents which are not always tolerated by IC patients.* Diaphragms can cause bladder (and vaginal) infections, because of the pressure placed on the bladder neck. The spermicide or lubricating jelly can also cause burning and spasms. Women with IC may be more comfortable and experience fewer side effects if their partner wears a condom. However, both male and female IC patients should avoid pre-lubricated condoms, those that contain spermicides and those made of latex, if they experience latex sensitivity.

IC patients are usually sensitive to commercial lubricants and spermicides. Spermicides can be irritating to the bladder, vagina and penis. They can kill friendly bacteria, making both men and women more susceptible to infection. IC patients need to rely on their partners to use the least irritating birth control possible. Women with IC who already have children or women who don't plan to have a family may consider asking their male partners to have a vasectomy.

IC patients who are not sensitive to progesterone may be able to tolerate birth control pills.

Alternative Positions for Intercourse

Our natural instincts tell us to avoid pain. Since certain sexual positions can increase pain and pressure, most IC patients figure out that if they have control of position and timing they are more willing to have intercourse. Some women have their male partners enter from a low angle when using the missionary position in order not to irritate the urethra.

It's essential to find a comfortable angle for entry. Intercourse can set off muscle spasms in both male and female IC patients. Intercourse should begin thoughtfully and slowly to help muscles gradually relax. A partner's understanding and involvement in the process of making intercourse more comfortable can bring a couple closer.

Pain Control After Sexual Intercourse

Swelling of the genitalia naturally occurs after intercourse, but the IC patient can experience prolonged vasoconstriction and increased nerve activity. Using an ice pack can reduce swelling, stinging and irritation. Applying direct heat can increase vasoconstriction, inflammation and the risk of infection.

Some IC patients benefit from cleansing the pelvic area after intercourse; however, the stimulation of washing may be painful. Relaxing in a warm bath instead can help to reduce spasms and swelling without the friction of spot cleansing. Patients who suffer with stiff muscles or fibromyalgia (FMS) may also benefit from a warm bath after intercourse. Drinking a glass of water is often necessary to dilute concentrated urine, to help reduce burning of tissues and to wash away bacteria that can end up in the bladder after intercourse.

MANAGING OVERLAPPING CONDITIONS THAT CAN INTERFERE WITH SEXUAL ACTIVITY

Different conditions can cause painful sex. One condition is IC, but IC patients often have co-existing conditions, as well as adhesions and nerve damage from previous surgeries, injuries and infections that contribute to their pain during sexual activity.

Some IC patients even experience an allergic reaction to their partner's semen after intercourse.* Treatments and preventive measures for co-existing conditions may improve the particular condition, the possibility for more comfortable intercourse and sometimes relieve IC symptoms. But as with any new treatment, IC patients must be aware of the possibility of triggering IC symptoms.

Women may experience burning, urgency, frequency, and bladder pain the morning after intercourse. A condom is advised for prevention. Allergist Jonathan Bernstein offers information on this allergy. See Resources.

Chronic Urinary Tract Infections

A urinary tract infection (UTI) can be set off by sexual activity. In IC patients, bacteria may come into contact with sensitive nerves between the bladder wall and lining, causing contraction of smooth muscle, burning and frequency. Symptoms may be difficult to distinguish from the symptoms of IC. Patients who experience recurrent bladder infections, especially related to sexual intercourse, often benefit from taking an antibiotic after sex as a preventive measure.

Doctors familiar with their patients' UTIs will usually be able to prescribe a good antibiotic for prevention. Patients who suffer with bladder infections after sex and do not use prevention may go through a very uncomfortable period of guessing, self-diagnosing and wondering whether to call their doctors, or not. Or they may not get into many doctors' offices right away. Waiting can be very painful and puts too much responsibility on patients. Taking an antibiotic before urinalysis will interfere with the reading. Refrigerating a specimen will cause bacteria to multiply and interfere with the reading. IC patients who experience recurring infections after sexual activity need to plan prevention with their doctors and keep a medication on hand for pain management.

Prevention for patients with recurrent UTIs includes washing the pelvic area with mild soap before sexual activity and drying the genitalia thoroughly after washing or bathing. However, IC patients who experience recurrent infections or those with secondary conditions such as vulvodynia may do best by using a blow dryer on a cool setting instead of a towel.

Yeast Infections

Yeast can inflame the vaginal lining and can also travel up the urethra and irritate the bladder. Although yeast supposedly does not thrive in an acidic atmosphere, which is thought to be maintained with regular sexual activity, the IC patient often suffers with yeast problems after sex. Contact and friction during intercourse can irritate the IC patient's vaginal tissue and yeast infections can occur. *For information on treatment and prevention of yeast see Chapter Five.*

Vulvodynia

Vulvodynia is a chronic condition which causes vulvar discomfort and pain. The symptoms of vulvodynia include irritation, itching, burning, pain, aching, throbbing, as well as a feeling of stretching or sucking-up. The pain and spasms cause an increase of histamines which leads to swelling, burning and itching. Patients experience sensitivity around the entrance to the vagina and painful sex. Patients with vulvodynia may also suffer with referred pain in the perineum, groin and buttocks, as well as the thighs and low back. Symptoms make sitting and walking difficult, and the pain and discomfort can keep patients up at night. Like IC, vulvodynia flares and responds to hormonal swings and menopause.

The different symptoms of vulvodynia are caused by various factors, and the condition is generally divided into two categories. Vulvodynia with a visible or known cause is considered *organic.* Vulvodynia with no visible abnormalities or known cause is considered *essential.* Organic vulvodynia is caused by factors such as chemical irritation, certain medications and invasive treatments, infections (including viral infections), nerve irritation, injury from laser treatment, and childbirth, etc.

Treatment varies for both categories of vulvodynia according to patients' particular symptoms, but treatment often includes yeast medications. Yeast can easily occur with, as well as cause irritated tissue. Estrogen cream is a standard treatment to prevent dry tissue from becoming susceptible to bacteria. Crisco shortening can also be used to soothe and prevent dryness of irritated vaginal tissue, but some IC patients may be sensitive to the ingredients. Topical anesthetics are sometimes prescribed for use during intercourse. Tricyclic antidepressants are prescribed in small doses to control symptoms and aid sleep. Anti-bacterial and anti-viral medications are also used. Some patients are treated with electrical stimulation either with a vaginal probe or small pads placed on their pelvic floor. Other patients are helped by pelvic floor massage therapy. These therapies are offered in some physical therapy clinics. *See Chapter One and Chapter Four.* In severe cases of vulvodynia, vestibular glands are sometimes removed.

Similar to the treatments for IC, the treatments for vulvodynia help some patients and not others, and may trigger a flare-up of symptoms. Oral medications can contain ingredients that aggravate the condition. Topical creams and ointments often contain substances, such as propylene glycol, sulfates, alcohol, and fragrance which have been known to irritate the condition of vulvodynia, as well as IC.

Vulvodynia patients may have problems with their bladders or have IC. One expression of vulvodynia that appears to be somewhat common in IC patients is vulvar vestibulitis. Vulvar vestibulitis is an inflammation of the glands that surround the vaginal entrance. Small red areas are the hallmark of this painful condition. Vulvar symptoms include itching, burning, sensitivity, shooting pains, and a tight, drawing feeling.

Because the conditions of IC, vulvodynia and FMS often overlap, researchers are studying the relationship of these diseases.

Patients who have both IC and vulvodynia should use a moderate approach to treatment. Pain management and prevention of vulvodynia symptoms include ice therapy, double rinsing underwear to remove excess soap, rinsing the irritated skin often with plain water (some patients use a squirt bottle), and as with IC, following a special diet. The foods known to trigger symptoms in vulvodynia are high in oxalates. These foods include many fruits and vegetables, nuts, some beverages, and grains which are believed to disturb the normal acid-base balance in the urine, and therefore, aggravate the vulvodynia. IC patients may feel challenged when trying to eliminate another list of foods. Fortunately, IC patient and author Bev Laumann offers recipes that are low in oxalates as well as bladder-safe in *A Taste of the Good Life*. *See Chapter Two*. Also available is *The Low Oxalate Diet Book* which can be ordered through the Vulvar Pain Foundation. *See Resources in Chapter One*.

Another approach to prevention of vulvodynia symptoms is taking calcium citrate supplements without vitamin D. Although some vulvodynia patients with IC have reported that taking the supplements has helped both their IC and vulvodynia symptoms, IC patients who are sensitive to many supplements may not be able to tolerate calcium citrate.

Endometriosis

Endometriosis is not typically associated with IC but there are many IC patients who must deal with both conditions. With endometriosis, fragments of endometrium tissue (from the lining of the uterus) travel from the uterus into the abdominal cavity where they can implant on the various pelvic organs. The fragments of tissue respond to the menstrual cycle and can grow and affect the area where they are located. When the fragments adhere to the bladder and/or intestines they can cause swelling and pain during elimination and urination. Endometrial fragments may also adhere to the supporting ligaments of the uterus, to surgical scars and even the chest cavity lining. Occasionally ovarian cysts are the result of endometriosis.

Patients with endometriosis may experience spotting, abnormal periods or heavy bleeding, pelvic and low back pain, painful intercourse, problems with colon activity and infertility. Endometriosis can cause internal scarring and may increase IC symptoms, especially during sexual intercourse and exercise.

A laparoscope is used to diagnose endometriosis. A biopsy is taken if endometrial tissue is not clearly recognizable. During a laparoscopy visible endometrium tissue can be eliminated with laser or with electrocautery. Although these procedures are often helpful, they are temporary and may trigger IC symptoms during the healing process. Most doctors turn to routine treatments first, such as combined birth control pills, progestins (synthetic progesterone) and induced menopause. However, these treatments can also set off IC symptoms which are not always temporary. Many IC patients cannot tolerate progestins or the progestational agents in birth control pills, and may suffer from the lack of estrogen with induced menopause. If endometriosis is very severe and a hysterectomy is necessary, estrogen replacement therapy is usually considered a common course of treatment. Of course, treatment will depend on the individual IC patient's reaction to estrogen.

Sjögren's Syndrome

Some IC patients have a chronic inflammatory condition called Sjögren's syndrome. Sjögren's syndrome causes excessive dryness in the secretory glands throughout the body. It is thought to be an autoimmune disease, has no known cause and mostly affects women. Also known as sicca syndrome, a dry mouth and dry eyes are considered the hallmark symptoms of this disease. Dryness and inflammation can affect other mucous membrane linings, such as the lining of the gastrointestinal tract, trachea, vulva and vagina. The lack of saliva in the mouth can lead to cavities, difficulty swallowing, and a lack of taste and smell. Cornea damage can occur because of a lack of tears and dry tissue in the vagina can lead to irritation, sometimes resulting in infection. Organs may also be affected in some patients.

Most women with Sjögren's syndrome are middle-aged. Symptoms of menopause usually make estrogen replacement, including topical estrogen, necessary. Proper lubrication, and warming-up pelvic muscles slowly before sexual activity are recommended.

DEALING WITH SEX AND YOUR PARTNER

Sex can enhance the quality of life, but if your last experience was painful, it's a normal reaction to avoid intercourse or even thinking about sex. However, it can be all too easy to let time slip by and not address sexual issues with your partner. When sexual issues aren't addressed they can contribute to intimacy avoidance, and lead to tension and fighting. The nature of the illness can make both you and your partner feel guilty: You, for not wanting sex and your partner for feeling demanding or selfish when he or she knows you are in pain. Feelings can be confusing and emotional, causing communication to break down. Your partner can easily feel rejected, but so can you even when you are the one saying *no*.

Aside from painful intercourse there may be another problem that interferes with sexual activity. Along with the symptoms of IC often comes a swollen belly and/or muscles that have gotten out-of-shape. Some IC patients may have a difficult time feeling desirable. Although a number of different factors go into one's self-image, self-image influences sexuality. Feeling attractive can be a challenge. This is why it is essential for IC patients to take as much control of their bodies as possible. First comes IC treatment and pain prevention. Next comes control of the whole body through gentle stretching and exercise. Even if medications add body weight and negative feelings, taking a little routine exercise every day or so will help to add strength, release tension and negative feelings, and build self-esteem. Self-nurturing also includes eating healthy foods, indulging in new clothes, furniture, plants, and make-up, or participating in activities that promote feelings of wholeness and confidence.

Although your partner might not always show it, IC pain has an effect on him or her, too. However, a partner who chooses to ignore your pain makes it difficult for you to demonstrate affection. Natural bonding and intimacy can suffer, because everyone needs touch and care. In order to get a relationship back on track you may have to show a little spontaneity and take advantage of the times when you feel better. Although you may have difficulty being spontaneous and deserve to have your pain and needs recognized, surprising a partner with a favorite dinner, a back rub or reservations at a favorite restaurant can be very reassuring, and recreate the necessary bonding that keeps relationships alive.

If a relationship has suffered, a good marriage counselor can help. A strong marriage can survive IC and IC can strengthen a good relationship. If a partner leaves a relationship and blames IC, there were probably other problems in the first place.

Dealing with Sex and a New Lover

Our youth oriented society seems to be defined by sexuality. Sex is everywhere and everyone is influenced. The younger IC patient must mature quickly, accept limitations, assume responsibility and be realistic about who she or he is and who she or he will become. It is important for a young person with IC to be protective when first getting to know someone special. There is no need to explain problems until one is sure that the other person is sincere and mature. Having IC does not have to keep a person from being desirable or intimate. If a new partner is understanding and willing to be pro-active, helps with pain management, prepares cold packs or whatever, you have a team player.

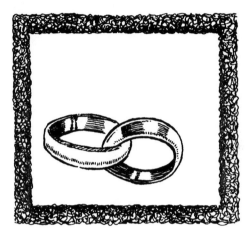

IC and Younger Couples

When IC strikes the younger couple who are just beginning a life together the effects can be quite different from those who have been together for a time. What the relationship is based on will determine how it can handle the illness. If a couple are good friends and communicative they probably will be able to work through any sexual issues. They can develop a very strong bond, and if they choose to start a family they can probably do so with a strong commitment.

IC, HORMONES, AND MID-LIFE CHANGES IN WOMEN

IC is not considered a progressive disease. Some research has shown that the symptoms of IC reach their peak and level off after about five years, yet symptoms still can and do change with the hormonal swings in women during their menstrual cycle, during pregnancy and during menopause. One survey of female IC patients reported that about 45 percent experienced their first IC symptoms after having a hysterectomy. Although men with IC also experience hormonal changes that affect their prostate and bladder symptoms, their hormones stay fairly steady until they age. Because there is not yet much information available on IC, men and hormones, this section will focus on the role of hormones in women with IC.

Research shows that hormonal changes affect systemic conditions with flare-ups and remissions, such as IC, FMS and chronic fatigue syndrome (CFS), vulvodynia, MCS, irritable bowel syndrome (IBS), Sjögren's syndrome and lupus. Migraines, yeast infections and other conditions are also triggered by hormonal swings, especially during perimenopause. Until recently, many illnesses and chronic conditions mostly prevalent in women have been blamed on psychological causes. Also, until quite recently hormone research has mainly been applied to male patients. Today, however, hormone research in women is a big topic offering new information almost daily.

Hormonal Changes During the Menstrual Cycle

The first day of the menstrual period is also day one of the menstrual cycle. Although both estrogen and progesterone are at their lowest levels on day one, estrogen begins to rise and continues to rise after menstruation. The rise in estrogen levels thickens the uterus in preparation for fertilization. The rise in estrogen also thickens the bladder lining during this time. Estrogen levels reach their peak at ovulation, at about day 14 of the cycle.

During the first two weeks of the menstrual cycle only a small amount of progesterone is present. However, after the egg is released during ovulation, estrogen levels quickly decline and progesterone levels begin to rise in preparation for pregnancy. Although estrogen levels also begin to rise again, they stay at a lower level than that of the first half of the menstrual cycle. During this second half of the menstrual cycle estrogen and progesterone levels reach a peak at around the same time, about the third week after the menstrual cycle. If the egg released during ovulation has been fertilized the progesterone levels remain high. If the egg has not been fertilized both the progesterone and estrogen production diminish quickly. The decline of progesterone levels causes the shedding of the endometrium, (the uterine lining) which begins a new menstrual cycle.

IC and the Menstrual Cycle

There is no set pattern for IC patients. There are patients who experience an increase in swelling, pressure, pain, and frequency when estrogen levels are highest. This is believed to happen because estrogen increases bladder mast cell secretion, therefore increasing inflammatory reactions. During this time IC patients may help to reduce their symptoms by avoiding fermented, and hot or spicy foods that increase histamine activity.

There are IC patients who feel better when their estrogen levels are high. They experience more comfortable intercourse, can eat more varied foods with less irritation, and have more energy. Experts believe that IC patients may benefit from the increase in the thickness of the bladder lining and the lack of progesterone during this time.

Some IC patients say they feel best and experience less IC symptoms during their menstrual period when hormone levels are low. However, other patients experience bladder pain during their periods, and almost all IC patients complain of IC symptoms a few days prior to the onset of bleeding. A number of IC patients also report pain just after a period and/or around ovulation. Experts may disagree about the effects hormones have on the IC bladder, but what they consistently agree upon is that the bladders of IC patients react to the rise and fall of hormone levels.

IC and PMS (premenstrual syndrome)

PMS occurs during the second half of the menstrual cycle when progesterone levels are at their highest. Common symptoms include fluid retention, irritability, headaches, backache, and sometimes abdominal pain. The lower estrogen levels and high progesterone levels make some IC patients more susceptible to bladder symptoms.

Patients with chronic conditions may also experience fatigue, stiff muscles, abdominal pressure and constipation when bowel activity slows down during this time. Sensitivities to the environment and to certain drugs may also be intensified during PMS. IC patients can try to reduce bladder symptoms by following a diet for IC, avoiding salt, sugar, caffeine, increasing fiber intake, eating small meals frequently (instead of three large meals), and engaging in some form of gentle exercise.

Perimenopause and Menopause

Perimenopause, sometimes referred to as "the climacteric," begins when a woman's estrogen levels start to decline. This decline usually begins in a woman's late 30's or early 40's, however, a few women can begin to experience perimenopausal symptoms in their early 30's. The average length of perimenopause is five to ten years.

Menopause (the cessation of periods) is believed to occur between the age of 45 and 55, with the average age at 51. Menopause can happen quickly or take two to four years. When a woman has had no menstrual period for 12 months and blood tests confirm the decline of estrogen, menopause is considered official. A woman is no longer in perimenopause. Instead, she is now in postmenopause. A woman who has her ovaries removed with hysterectomy has what is called surgical menopause.

Symptoms During Perimenopause

Symptoms vary woman to woman because the approach to menopause is so individual. Fluctuations of estrogen create hormonal swings which in turn can cause night sweats, waking episodes, insomnia, hot flashes, chills, palpitations, lighter, heavier, or irregular periods, complexion problems, depression, and troubles with memory and concentration. Women in early perimenopause can experience lighter periods, night sweats, insomnia, painful PMS, and constipation. As hormone levels continue to drop, symptoms can change. Blood tests are used to determine hormone levels.

Physical Changes that Affect the Bladder During Perimenopause

All women experience change in their bladders and vaginas during menopause. Elizabeth Lee Vliet, M.D., writes in her book *Screaming To Be Heard*, of the many direct effects estrogen has on the bladder lining, as well as the nerves, blood vessels, and muscles that govern urinary function. She explains that the smooth muscle in the bladder, urethra and vagina lose tone and strength as estrogen levels decline. This decline in estrogen concurrently increases sensitivity to pain and susceptibility to bladder problems.

When there is a decrease in blood flow and lubrication, the urethral, bladder and vaginal tissue become thinner, drier, less resilient, and more susceptible to inflammation. Supporting muscles and tissue of the bladder and uterus lose tone and stability, allowing the bladder to fall downward. The dropping of the bladder can change the angle of the urethra making the bladder more susceptible to outside bacteria. These various changes leave the bladder vulnerable to infection and can cause symptoms such as urgency, frequency, burning, and sometimes mild incontinence (IC does not lead to or cause incontinence). Women who suffer with chronic urethral pressure, frequency and other bladder symptoms may be diagnosed with urethral syndrome. Urethral syndrome is sometimes treated with bladder dilation. Dilation should be avoided because it can cause scarring, injury and incontinence, as well as worsen the symptoms of IC, even if IC is experienced later.

As IC patients begin to reach menopause their IC symptoms can also change. Patients who are used to feeling relief upon urination (due to the lack of blood flow when voiding) may experience some burning in their urethra instead. Patients in early perimenopause may begin to notice cramping in their pelvic floor around ovulation, right before or after their menstrual period. Patients who also have endometriosis, or IBS may experience more pain from inflammation and built-up scar tissue as hormones begin to decline. In general, women with injured muscles and ligaments from surgeries, childbirth or low back problems may experience compounded weakness and bladder problems. Pressure on pelvic veins can cause painful varicose veins, pelvic and leg pain. Perimenopause is a time to keep back muscles strong, use good support while sitting and avoid lifting heavy objects.

Coping with IC and Other Conditions
During Perimenopause

Many patients are in perimenopause when diagnosed with IC. It's easy to comprehend the challenge of a chronic condition during perimenopause. Symptoms such as disturbed sleep, palpitations, constipation, fatigue, muscle pain, and weakness are often intensified at this time. Determining which symptoms are part of perimenopause and which are part of the chronic illness may be difficult and confusing. However, symptoms should not be ignored. Women in general must begin to listen to their bodies more closely, and IC patients may need to be aware of common overlapping conditions that may occur during perimenopause.

Heart palpitations may be a natural symptom of perimenopause and may sometimes be uncomfortable for IC patients with mitral valve prolapse (MVP). However, palpitations can also indicate a heart condition or more often in IC patients, a thyroid disorder. Thyroid production decreases as one ages and women who experience irregular and run-away periods, fatigue, heart palpitations and anxiety attacks, as well as, painful PMS should ask their doctors for a thyroid function test. This test should be done along with hormone levels tested during perimenopause, because it is not unusual for IC and FMS patients to also have hypothyroidism, low functioning thyroid.

Estrogen enhances thyroid replacement, and may also be needed during perimenopause. If thyroid levels turn out to be borderline and doctors do not want to prescribe thyroid medication, IC patients should ask for a repeat test. If there is no change and patients cannot get treatment for symptoms, it's time to see other doctors. Patients with chronic illnesses who test borderline, or close to, often need treatment even if the doctor does not agree. Patients with irregular periods who are given birth control pills as treatment should be aware that they can aggravate bladder symptoms.

IC patients who suffer with fatigue and shakiness may also want to ask to be tested for anemia or pernicious anemia (B12 deficiency). Pernicious anemia appears to affect patients with chronic conditions.

Inflammations and infections in the vagina and bladder that occur with hormone changes are more difficult to treat for patients with IC, vulvodynia, Sjögren's syndrome, CFS, IBS and patients with chronic yeast infections. Natural fatigue during perimenopause can be more challenging. Patients with migraine headaches, drug, and environmental sensitivities may also become more vulnerable to their symptoms.

It's obvious that a woman with a chronic illness feels less in control during perimenopause. The IC patient used to predicting and understanding her symptoms by her menstrual cycle will have to readjust. Menopause can be very stressful. The IC patient may have to work more closely with her urologist or gynecologist or find a urogynecologist. Estrogen replacement and/or new treatments and medications may be needed to control symptoms. It's important to realize that when periods start up, become somewhat regular, then stop again, new symptoms of IC that may accompany perimenopause can also change. Some do get better or even go away. The experience of menopause is not a final sentence. It's a time when the healthy peers of an IC patient also must slow down and pay attention to their bodies.

Estrogen Replacement for IC and General Health

Studies have shown estrogen helps women to control cholesterol levels and keep bones strong.* Estrogen stimulates cell growth and proliferation which helps the skin and arteries. Estrogen also enhances thyroid production, assists memory and concentration and may as well help to reduce the risk of Alzheimer's disease and colon cancer. There are however, risks involved with estrogen replacement therapy (ERT) which will be discussed later in this chapter.

Estrogen plays a role in the management of many chronic conditions. The effects of estrogen seem to fight pain in a variety of conditions. Many IC patients avoid severe bladder, muscle and joint pain and IBS symptoms with estrogen replacement.

Studies are ongoing to understand estrogen's role in preventing heart disease.

Hormone Replacement Choices

There are standard blood tests to determine hormone levels and the appropriate dose of hormone replacement, but finding the right time to begin replacement and the correct level or type of hormone replacement is often "trial by error" for patients with

IC. IC patients need to work with gynecologists or naturopaths who specialize in alternative medication (if using estrogen supplements) to regulate hormonal balance, because everything changes during menopause, including IC.

No matter how supportive a doctor is of hormone replacement, he or she may not realize the full impact of hormones in IC patients. Doctors may not be aware that there are IC patients who cannot tolerate estrogen that is opposed with progesterone, but usually will understand if their patients explain that progesterone increases symptoms in women with other conditions, such as migraine headaches. However, there is a conflict of opinions about the symptoms and benefits of progesterone today. Many of those who promote natural plant progesterone cream blame the imbalance of progesterone and estrogen during perimenopause as the cause of PMS and menopausal symptoms. According to this belief, during menopause progesterone production can become irregular and leave estrogen unopposed. The unopposed estrogen is then believed to cause the symptoms of PMS, hot flashes, bloating, insomnia, depression, and irregular periods. Some supporters of this theory believe that even the phytoestrogens in your diet must be balanced. Alternative doctors and naturopaths usually promote natural progesterone, but they also may vary in their theories and treatments.

The other school of thought (which usually consists of doctors who practice traditional medicine) is that progesterone is the cause of PMS, bloating, constipation, insomnia, headaches, and depression. Hot flashes and irregular periods are blamed on the decline of estrogen during perimenopause, and progestins (synthetic progesterone) taken to oppose estrogen during HRT (hormone replacement therapy) are blamed as the cause of constipation and bloating (unopposed estrogen appears to help with regularity).

The doctor a woman sees can determine her hormone replacement therapy. So can a woman's health, because there are risks involved when replacing estrogen. The most active form of estrogen, estradiol (the estrogen routinely prescribed), is capable of causing growth of the uterus and breasts, as well as vaginal and other estrogen-sensitive tissues, such as the bladder. Your doctor must evaluate your personal health profile, as well as your family history when prescribing hormone replacement therapy. Because estrogen increases the risk of cell build up in the lining of the uterus, a woman is usually prescribed estrogen opposed with progesterone, especially those with endometriosis. If the IC patient chooses unopposed estrogen to relieve bladder symptoms, her doctor may suggest a pap smear twice a year and an edometrial biopsy if she experiences bleeding. The IC patient with endometriosis can have a difficult time making choices as her estrogen levels fall.

As always, what works depends on the individual IC patient. There are some IC patients who cannot tolerate estrogen or progesterone. And there are some IC patients who can use plant supplements. The following information reviews some of the available hormone replacement choices. Each IC patient must make an informed decision based on her IC and the advice of her doctor. It's helpful to read as much as possible and stay abreast of new forms of hormone replacement and new IC treatments.

Progesterone Choices

Progestogens include synthetic progestins (including designer progesterone) and natural progesterone. Natural progesterone is derived from plants, soy and wild yams, and so far is used most effectively to reduce the risk of endometrial cancer when taken in a prescription capsule or vaginal gel. (Vaginal gels may cause burning and irritation in IC patients.) Both natural progesterone and progestins produce a similar anti-growth factor in the uterus like that of the body's own progesterone. Until recently, doctors have been skeptical about the effectiveness of natural progesterone. They either considered it too weak to treat menopausal symptoms and prevent health risks, or too strong for unregulated, self-medication.

Doctors or naturopaths who promote natural progesterone support the theory that it doesn't provoke the side effects of synthetic progestins, such as headaches, bloating, and weight gain. Also, they find that unlike progestin, natural progesterone does not interfere as severely with the benefits of estrogen, such as prevention of heart disease. Some promoters of natural progesterone suggest it may actually reduce the risks of heart disease and counteract the risks of breast cancer that is usually associated with long-term estrogen use. However, more evidence is needed and according to the *Harvard Women's Health Watch* (October 1999), women should be aware that the benefits of progesterone creams may be overrated.

Progestogens in general seem to be poorly tolerated by a number of IC patients. Plant progesterones are known to increase urinary frequency in women without IC.

Estrogen Choices

The available various estrogens work differently and offer different benefits. Estradiol is usually a doctor's choice of estrogen replacement for women beginning hormone replacement therapy. Estradiol is the predominant natural human estrogen most abundantly produced by the ovaries before menopause. Estradiol is also the form of estrogen that occurs naturally in plants according to the *Harvard Women's Health Watch* (December 1998).

Today there are several choices and many ways to use estrogen replacement: a vaginal or topical cream, oral medication, skin patch, injection, or implant. However, most doctors like to prescribe the oral tablet Premarin. According to Elizabeth Lee Vliet, M.D., in *Screaming To Be Heard*, "Many doctors consider that Premarin is the 'gold standard' for estrogen therapy because it is the one which has been on the market longer, and most of the research studies have used only this one type of estrogen to determine estrogen benefits, side effects, and risks" (p. 97). Premarin has been subject to more debate in recent years as the reported number of side effects have increased.

Phytoestrogens (plant estrogens) are available in prescription drugs as well as through drug and healthfood stores. Plant estrogens that are not prescription are defined as supplements because they are not FDA approved. Phytoestrogens are available in transdermal patches, pills and creams. Estrogen creams are available through formulating pharmacies that make custom-tailored hormone replacement. One such company that also makes a topical pain gel for chronic pain patients is New England Formulating Pharmacy. *See Resources in Chapter Five.**

New drugs called designer estrogens imitate estrogen, but have the ability to block the effects of estrogen in parts of the body where it's not needed, such as in the breast. Estrogen receptors are located in the bones, breast, uterus, urogenital system, and the brain. Patients with certain conditions or a hereditary predisposition to certain conditions must avoid estrogen that can adversely affect these areas.

If the IC patient cannot find the right hormone replacement she can consult a reproductive endocrinologist to problem-solve.

Estrogen Cream

Some IC patients control the early symptoms of menopause with estrogen cream which can be applied topically on the belly, thighs, vulva, or inserted vaginally. The effects of the different estrogen creams are very individual, but in general they appear not to deliver the consistent dose or systemic benefits of other forms of estrogen. This can be both good and bad, depending on the patients' needs, age and risks factors.

The effectiveness of estrogen creams inserted vaginally also depends on the condition of the vaginal lining and thickness of the vaginal wall. Evidence so far shows that estrogen creams help to alleviate some vulvar and vaginal symptoms, such as dryness, itching and burning with urination, and may help to prevent bladder infections. However, creams applied close to the uterus have in some instances stimulated endometrial proliferation.

There are IC patients who use estrogen creams during perimenopause until they need a stronger estrogen. Some patients continue to use a little estrogen cream topically for vulvar and urethral symptoms after they begin a stronger estrogen. Estrogen cream alone does not appear to help very much with IC symptoms, but does appear to help some women prevent certain vulvar and urethral symptoms.

Estrogen creams in general contain inactive ingredients that may irritate the bladder, urethra and the vulva. Patients complain of reactions to propylene glycol, alcohol and fragrance, however, there are IC patients who find the estrogen cream Estrace tolerable. But, as usual, IC patients should always try a small amount of any new cream away from the urethra. *See Estrogen Choices in this chapter.*

Oral Estrogen

Prescription oral estrogen can be animal or plant based. Most women are prescribed the oral supplement Premarin. Some IC patients do well with Premarin. Yet IC patients who also have IBS may find that they do not get the consistent full benefit of oral estrogen because of poor bowel absorption (oral estrogen must go through the digestive tract which actually offers benefits to those who absorb it properly). IC patients may also experience bladder pain and other reactions to the dyes and inactive ingredients in the different brands of oral estrogen, or to particular estrogens. Some women have reported muscle spasms and leg cramping thought to be triggered by equine estrogen (pregnant mares' urine).

Since medications are very challenging, the IC patient should begin with a low level estrogen at first. This is important unless there is severe bladder pain due to the lack of estrogen. In this case a strong dosage is usually necessary. The patient may have to switch brands if the first type of estrogen isn't agreeable or does not relieve her bladder symptoms. Also, if estrogen replacement is started before needed, the IC patient can experience a negative reaction.

Estrogen Patch

Many IC patients prefer to use an estrogen patch. There is less hormone needed with a patch because the estrogen and inactive ingredients do not have to be broken down in the stomach and intestines as oral estrogen does. Instead they flow through the skin into the bloodstream. Patches contain adhesives, membranes, gels, and protective films that may be irritating to patients with sensitive skin, chemical sensitivities and allergies. Estrogen and added ingredients in estrogen patches may also irritate the bladder.

Although prescription estrogen patches do not improve cholesterol levels as effectively as oral estrogen, they appear to relieve menopausal symptoms, help to prevent osteoporosis and relieve IC symptoms in many patients. Some IC patients find they can tolerate the prescription estrogen patch Viville, however, estrogen replacement is always individual.

An estrogen patch can be used at a low level during perimenopause and then switched to a higher level later, or whenever needed. Patients in perimenopause who experience bad migraines and/or IC symptoms just before their menses are sometimes helped by using an estrogen patch preventively during this time. Women who cannot tolerate estrogen replacement will usually know right away with symptoms of nervousness, headache, increased pelvic pressure, bladder discomfort, or pain.

Plant Estrogens

Prescription phytoestrogens contain components that are chemically synthesized from plant material, such as soy. These compounds are similar to the estrogens found in the body. Estrogen supplements are derived from dietary and herbal sources found in soy, flax, dong quoi, and black cohosh.

Promoters of estrogen supplements believe they have a good effect on cholesterol levels, fight osteoporosis, may act as anti-growth factors in the uterus, and fight breast and prostate cancer. Estrogen supplements also appear to reduce the surge of some hormones during mid-cycle. Those in favor of supplements believe that they do not pose a risk when taken in low doses without opposing progesterone. These claims are not conclusive and more research is needed.

Prescription plant estrogens are generally thought to present the same risks as Premarin when used without progesterone. However, prescription plant estrogens offer a consistent dose and do not deliver the unwanted properties and effects of herbal and plant supplements.

Designer Estrogens

New designer estrogens offer fewer dangerous side effects to women who are at high risk for breast cancer and other conditions. These estrogens are referred to as SERMS, selective estrogen-receptor modulators. They are supposed to offer the good qualities of estrogen and none of the bad, and are available to women who cannot take other forms of estrogen that may increase their individual health risks. SERMS increase bone density, decreasing the risks of osteoporosis, and heart attacks without posing a risk of breast cancer or uterine bleeding. SERMS do not control hot flashes, sleep disturbance and vaginal dryness. Because they do not cause growth in estrogen-sensitive tissues, such as the bladder lining, they probably will not help IC patients who depend on estrogen replacement for relief of IC symptoms.

Slow Release Estrogen

Most IC patients should probably avoid hormone implants and injections. Long lasting forms of slow release hormones cannot offer the same control and pain management of other forms of estrogen. Also, devices such as an estrogen ring which is inserted like a diaphragm and about the same size, are usually not comfortable for IC patients. The benefit of an estrogen ring is that it treats vaginal symptoms and maybe bladder symptoms without the same systemic effects of other methods.

Menopause Management
without Hormone Replacement

IC patients who cannot take estrogen must supplement their diet with calcium rich foods and some form of weight bearing exercise such as walking. Those who can should take calcium supplements and eat foods for their mineral, vitamin and estrogen properties. If women can tolerate soy products and/or flaxseed oil they may benefit by adding these dietary estrogens to their diet. Foods and oils that do not agree with IC patients when first tried should be avoided.

Vaginal dryness should be addressed to prevent inflammation and infection. Lubricants can help with prevention (*see Lubrication Choices in this chapter*) and some patients can use hydrocortisone creams to calm inflammation. However, hydrocortisone can be irritating to the bladder and should be tried very sparingly. IC patients who cannot tolerate estrogen and experience a worsening of symptoms with menopause may have to try new medications or follow a stricter diet to calm the bladder during and after menopause. Of course, there are women who feel better after menopause with no hormone replacement.

Postmenopause

Until recently, how long women took estrogen depended on their symptoms and what doctors were taught in medical school. Some women continued hormone replacement for two to five years after menopause. Some only took estrogen for a few months to control symptoms, and some women didn't take estrogen at all. Women who took estrogen were often advised to reduce their dosage after they had taken estrogen for a certain length of time. This was because it did not seem to be necessary and because of the increased risks of breast cancer after five to ten years. Now the connection between breast cancer and estrogen are being further investigated. For IC and other patients with chronic conditions, estrogen replacement may be needed for the rest of their lives.

The beliefs that have dictated estrogen therapy are changing. Estrogen is now recognized as important for the prevention and control of certain illnesses. New designer estrogens are available for high risk patients. More choices for estrogen therapy are available for the different needs of women. The future of hormone replacement appears hopeful, more sophisticated and safer.

Hormone replacement is still serious business. Hormones are very powerful. If a woman decides to reduce her dosage she should taper off slowly and alternate the higher dose (her present dose) with the lower dose every other day. If a woman wants to end her hormone therapy she also should taper off slowly. This is best done with a doctor's direction and the awareness that the IC patient should make any change very slowly.

Health Risks at Mid-Life

Doctors make evaluations at menopause and mid-life for both female and male patients. Tests and prevention for diseases that may be present at mid-life are becoming standardized. Middle-aged patients fall into a sort of "package treatment program" with insurance companies and doctors. Although IC does not exclude patients from their mid-life regime of tests and maintenance, there is now an excess in testing for women. According to the *Harvard Women's Health Watch* (April, 1998) "Women's health has (also) become a 'hot market.' As a result, we've been bombarded by promotional campaigns for new tests to detect certain diseases and some of these may be unnecessary" (p. 1).

The IC patient can work best with a primary care doctor who understands and works with her individual sensitivities to medicines, dyes and liquids used during certain tests. Referred specialists and technicians who evaluate and give tests may not know or understand IC.

IC patients may want to subscribe to the *Harvard Women's Health Watch* in order to receive the most updated information on women. Back issues can be ordered from an information sheet listing different topics and hormone options. *See Resources.*

For more information on hormones and how they affect women, including those with IC, read the book *Screaming To Be Heard* by Elizabeth Lee Vliet, M.D.

PREGNANCY AND IC

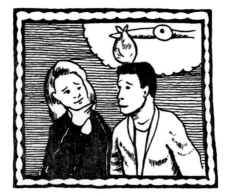

According to available information on pregnancy and IC, a large number of patients fall into the childbearing age bracket. Many patients give positive feedback when asked about their pregnancies. In a small study, IC mothers reported having no more difficulty becoming pregnant than women without IC. IC mothers also reported the same rate of deliveries and healthy babies as other women. Many women with IC have second babies and report that they feel better when they are pregnant. Some experts believe that women with chronic illnesses improve with pregnancy because of the changes in their immune systems.

Preparing for Pregnancy and IC

Every woman's goal is to have a healthy baby, but a woman with IC has the added goal of keeping her bladder symptoms under control during pregnancy. She quickly learns the key to success with IC and pregnancy is good planning.

Planning before conception may allow the IC patient to get symptoms under control before becoming pregnant. Learning alternative pain management for IC symptoms before conception is beneficial throughout pregnancy because bladder treatments and medicines should usually be discontinued. Pain management before conception may mean avoiding intercourse, except, of course, during ovulation.

Pain prevention and planning are not limited to preconception. IC management is helpful throughout pregnancy, delivery and child care, and can begin when the IC patient learns she is pregnant.

Support During Pregnancy

Physically, younger women may have an easier time with pregnancy. However, many IC patients, both young and older, find they feel better than usual when they are pregnant. But a good pregnancy depends on factors other than feeling physically well. Patients need the support and understanding of others, doctors who will listen, and if needed, the guidance of family counselors.

Networking with other IC patients can also be very helpful. The ICA offers a nationwide list of women who have been pregnant or who are currently pregnant. To order a list of patients send a self-addressed stamped envelope to the ICA with a pregnancy support list request. The IC Network offers up-to-date information, as well as a wonderful message board and chat room for questions and answers. *Refer to Resources in Chapter One.*

Picking the Right Doctor

A woman with IC may not qualify for special, or what is called *high risk* treatment, even when she does not comfortably fit into the routine approach. If a patient has developed a good relationship with her OB/GYN concerning IC, she may do best continuing with this doctor. However, if the IC patient feels that she may need medication during pregnancy or be intensely managed, the ICA suggests in its Treatment and Self-help brochure *IC and Pregnancy* that a woman may consider choosing an obstetrician who specializes in high risk pregnancy or urology. Of course, the woman with IC may still have to convince a new doctor of her unique needs.

The woman with IC may also want to ask for a thyroid function test along with her pregnancy test. The thyroid is directly linked with reproduction and hypothyroidism (thyroid deficiency) can interfere with conception, and can make pregnancy more difficult. It can take a repeat thyroid test to detect low thyroid levels. If you have trouble conceiving you may have to be persistent if you suspect that you have a thyroid deficiency.

If a fertility specialist is needed you will most probably be treated as other women without IC. Although you have to let your doctor know that IC pain management is a concern for you, the specialist might not be open or able to help you avoid some discomfort during fertility treatment. *See Elizabeth and Pregnancy in Chapter Ten.*

Bladder Changes during Pregnancy

Many patients report that they experience less bladder, muscle and joint pain than before pregnancy. Some experts believe that remission of symptoms during pregnancy occurs in many chronic pain patients because the immune system is suppressed during pregnancy. Female hormones regulate the immune processes in women. Bladder frequency and some of the other IC symptoms, however, are a part of pregnancy. This is especially true during the early and late part of pregnancy when there is extra pressure on the bladder.

IC patients who also have FMS may experience a worsening of their muscle symptoms during the last trimester. IC patients in general may experience the most relief during the middle trimester.

Pain Management during Pregnancy

As with the individual symptoms of each IC patient, every IC pregnancy is unique. Although the IC patient is usually familiar with her own pain triggers, pregnancy is a time to follow stricter guidelines for IC pain prevention to avoid prescription treatments or medications.

Options for pain management and treatment include a diet for IC, relaxation techniques, gentle exercise, massage therapy (only with a doctor's consent), and keeping to a routine daily schedule. The bladder is calmer when the IC patient feels in control and less stressed.

Medications during Pregnancy

Dealing with your bladder can be your biggest concern besides your baby, however, at times, there may be other minor conditions to deal with. You may be used to avoiding a variety of medications due to bladder sensitivity and you may use alternative treatments for minor illnesses and conditions, but during pregnancy it's necessary to work with the doctor to treat problems that arise. Self-medication, including over-the-counter medications should be avoided.

Even if a doctor prescribes a drug or an over-the-counter medication, it's a good idea to investigate the risks of all medications to avoid bladder pain, other sensitivities and of course, risks to the baby's health. It is also vital to make the doctor aware of every medication that you are taking or condition you are being treated for.

Diet and Pregnancy

Some IC patients experience bladder relief during pregnancy and find they can eat a greater variety of foods than before pregnancy. However patients should be aware that food tolerance can change with the hormonal changes of each trimester. Some patients need to be more disciplined during their third trimester and some must stick to a bladder-safe diet throughout pregnancy.

Nutrition and Prenatal Vitamins

Pregnant women are advised to take prenatal vitamins and eat nutrient-rich produce high in vitamins. Tolerating the food sources and vitamins that supply the needed nutrition during pregnancy can be a challenge for IC patients. Prenatal vitamins contain lots of vitamin C and B-6 which may trigger IC symptoms. Bev Laumann suggests a helpful strategy: Pregnant IC patients can write down the amounts of each vitamin listed on their prenatal vitamin bottles. Then they can buy the individual vitamins in the listed dosages. Naturally, patients should try one supplement at a time to detect tolerance. Some patients find they must avoid vitamins B-6 and C, although buffered C (with calcium carbonate) or the version called "ester C" are sometimes tolerated.

It's very important for IC patients to read up on nutrition and pregnancy. It's also necessary for patients to put a lot of color and different foods into their daily diet in order to get necessary vitamins and minerals. Some experts suggest that IC patients consult a nutritionist when there's uncertainty about meeting nutritional requirements. Understanding professionals may help IC patients to problem-solve, feel more supported and less worried which is best for mom and baby. *For information on alternative vitamin sources refer to the vitamin-rich foods suggested in Chapter Two and to the following information.*

Calcium

Adequate calcium is necessary during pregnancy. The IC patient who cannot tolerate calcium supplements must add extra calcium-rich foods, such as dairy products, to her diet. If dairy products are tolerable, the IC patient can drink milk, eat ricotta cheese (check for added vinegar), cottage cheese, cream cheese, and ice cream (the less additives in ice cream the better). Individuals with lactose intolerance can sometimes tolerate yogurt, which is a good source of calcium. Plain, vanilla or maple are usually best, because yogurt made with fruit contains more sugar and the fruit may be a bladder irritant.

Whole milk dairy products provide a better source of calcium than skim or low fat dairy products, because fat enhances calcium absorption. If a pregnant woman is restricted to low fat dairy products, she should eat her main source of daily calcium along with another food that contains fat. For example, she can have a glass of low fat milk with a piece of buttered toast, or with a salad dressed in olive oil or another oil based dressing. A salad with a plain yogurt and oil dressing is also a good source of calcium.

Other rich sources of calcium can be found in salmon and tofu, if tolerated. It's important to avoid foods like spinach and other dark greens when eating your main calcium source. Although these foods offer a good source of iron and other nutrients they can decrease calcium absorption. Eating too much fiber while consuming a main source of calcium can also rob the body of needed calcium.

Iron

Foods and supplements rich in iron are very important during pregnancy. Unfortunately, not all IC patients can tolerate iron supplements and need to eat foods that supply a good source of iron, such as beef, beef liver and other meats, poultry, fish, egg yolks, and kidney and baked beans (preferably not in tomato sauce). Nuts, if tolerated, also provide a source of iron and other minerals. Just a small handful of nuts can supply patients with a lot of nutrition. Some IC patients say that they can eat cashews, pine nuts and almonds. Some patients can tolerate hazel, Brazil nuts, pecans, and peanuts.

Iron is more easily absorbed when eaten with foods that are rich in vitamin C. Most IC patients cannot tolerate orange juice and other citrus fruits. However, they can eat potatoes and other produce rich in vitamin C along with meat, poultry and fish which are the best absorbed sources of iron. *Refer to Chapter Two for produce rich in vitamin C.*

Adequate fiber is very important during pregnancy, especially when taking iron supplements which can provoke constipation. There are different iron supplements available for those who have this problem. There are also alternative supplements available for patients who are sensitive to iron, such as iron drops for babies and vitamin supplements for children. Of course, these sources of iron may need to be taken more often for adults to benefit.

B Vitamins

Taking B vitamins before conception can help prepare the body for pregnancy. B vitamins are extremely important throughout pregnancy and during lactation. They help the body utilize key nutrients and work best when taken together, as in a B-complex supplement or a multivitamin, such as a prenatal supplement.

If B vitamins are irritating, they can be consumed alternatively in liver, whole and unrefined grains, brown rice, leafy vegetables, milk and eggs, fortified foods and cereals (if tolerated). *See Chapter Two for more information on B vitamins.*

Stress and Pregnancy

The IC patient is used to controlling the stress in her life in order to keep symptoms quiet. Pregnancy is the time to take even more control, because stress causes the release of certain chemicals in the body. These chemicals can affect both a baby's physical and emotional health. Extra stress can be avoided by living with a regular schedule and sleeping pattern, as well as practicing stress reduction exercises. New findings show that a baby seems to adjust to people and situations better when the mother keeps to a regular schedule during pregnancy.

With more focus on prenatal care and stress prevention, helpful information is being researched. Although some facts are just common sense, experiments and data now support these claims with scientific evidence to further support a pregnant woman and her baby. The effects of stress and the different types of stress that may occur during pregnancy are being studied. For example, a study on the effects of music on a fetus showed that soft music is very good for a baby while loud music is not. When loud music was aimed at a mother's abdomen the fetus actually urinated. Another study demonstrated a common stress: working pregnant women are often placed under additional work demands as they prepare to take their maternity leave. Reading current research and information on pregnancy can provide valuable information and guidelines.

Exercise and Good Body Mechanics

Pregnancy is a time to try to stay strong and flexible. Some IC patients feel better than usual and are, therefore, more motivated to exercise. However, pregnancy is not the time for patients to take on new forms of challenging exercise. IC patients may be susceptible to muscle and/or bladder pain from too many repetitions of an exercise, holding a position for too long, over-stretching muscles, and/or performing jarring movements. Trying to keep up with other pregnant women who do not have IC should not be a goal. Comfort and avoidance of fatigue should be a goal.

Following recommended gentle exercise to increase flexibility and strengthen the neck and lower back muscles can help IC patients carry their babies during and after pregnancy. Strength and flexibility in these areas are especially important in late-stage pregnancy when the extra weight and shift in the pelvis change the body's balance. Changes in the lower body affect the legs and feet, and leave the upper body with less support (most IC patients already have some compromise in their lower body due to the muscle weakness in their pelvic region). Women in general may experience fatigue, fluid retention, leg cramps and pressure, including pressure in the pelvic floor. Cramping in the feet and legs can often be relieved with regular flexion, extension and rotation exercises of the feet. Calcium supplements and/or calcium-rich foods can also help to control cramping in the legs and feet. Walking and/or swimming can improve circulation.

Always talk to a doctor before beginning any new exercise regime and be aware of exercises and movements that should be avoided as pregnancy progresses. Don't wait until the last trimester to begin an exercise regime. A patient with low back problems before pregnancy should inform her doctors, because she may become vulnerable to cystitis especially when her body's balance changes. Low back strengthening is often prescribed. Strengthening in general and following the suggestions in *Chapter Three* can be helpful. Be sure to consult your doctor first.

Kegel Exercise

Women are sometimes advised to prepare their pelvic floor for delivery with Kegel exercises. Kegel exercises are intended to help women strengthen and improve voluntary control over their pelvic muscles. Not all IC patients can contract their pelvic floor muscles or start and stop their urine stream without pain. Many IC patients must avoid stopping a urine stream because voiding can bring relief and interruption can interfere. Kegel exercises are also related to orgasm. Doctors and therapists may promote the benefits of Kegel to their patients both sexually and preventively, but performing pelvic floor exercises is often not possible without triggering pelvic floor pain.

Pelvic floor exercises to strengthen the supporting muscles of the bladder and urethra are also prescribed to control incontinence that sometimes occurs with pregnancy. Pelvic floor strengthening may, or may not work for incontinence during pregnancy, but incontinence usually goes away after delivery. If the IC patient uses Kegel exercise, she should keep her abdominal muscles relaxed when tightening her pelvic floor muscles. She should also avoid holding her breath. If Kegel exercises are agreeable, they should begin before the last trimester, if possible.

Massage and Muscle Therapy During Pregnancy

Some IC patients just feel better all over with the hormones during pregnancy. However, many pregnant women can benefit from massage and muscle therapy. Gentle "bodywork" or massage can help to prevent tension, discourage muscles from shortening, encourage circulation, and reduce fluid retention, all of which may add to muscle and bladder pain in IC patients. Of course, it is important to discuss any type of hands-on therapy with a doctor before pursuing this option.

During the last trimester some women with IC and other chronic conditions experience an increase in muscle pain and even the best therapies may not be as helpful as before.

177

Following the general advice for pain relief, such as wearing support hose, using good ergonomics (supporting both the upper and lower back while sitting) and avoiding shoes or sandals with a negative heel can help to distribute body weight more evenly and provide better support.

Urinary Tract Infections

Hormonal changes during pregnancy cause the muscle tone of the urinary system to relax. At the same time, hormonal changes cause the kidneys to produce more urine. These physical changes in bladder function make a woman more vulnerable to bladder infections. Experts suggest that the IC patient have a urinalysis each prenatal visit. There are two factors that can contribute to an undetected urinary tract infection. First, the IC patient may have difficulty distinguishing IC symptoms from those of a bladder infection, and second, the pregnant woman doesn't always feel the symptoms of an infection. If there's ever any question of infection, it's vital to contact the doctor. Infected urine can affect the baby.

Naturally, no one wants to take antibiotics during pregnancy, and for the IC patient, antibiotics can mean bladder pain, frequency, yeast infections, and other allergic reactions. If you are prone to bladder infections it may be advisable to establish a plan and discuss antibiotic treatment with your doctor in the beginning of pregnancy. This can help to avoid explanation and perhaps conflict later if there is an infection.

Larrian Gillespie suggests that it becomes more difficult to get a clean urine specimen further into pregnancy. As a woman becomes larger she sits with her buttocks and pelvis rolled back and under in a posterior position due to the extra weight carried in the front of the body. It's believed that catching a urine specimen in this position can cause urine to run back into the vagina and, therefore, contaminate the catch. Using an alternative position while voiding may help a woman to get a cleaner catch and void more completely. To find an alternative position while sitting, sit as far back on the toilet seat as possible, lifting your buttocks up in the back and opening your legs out so you can lean forward. This seated posture brings the upper body forward over the pelvis, allowing abdominal muscles to rest and the bladder to empty more fully and more directly into the specimen bottle. If a urine catch tests positive for infection ask to give another specimen to double check. The doctor can also confirm infection with a catheter specimen.

Yeast Infections
The normal acid environment of the vagina changes as vaginal secretions increase during pregnancy. These changes contribute to yeast infections. Using prevention with diet by reducing sweets and refined carbohydrates may help to reduce yeast in the large intestine where it can flourish with constipation. Prevention also includes staying dry, wearing skirts and cotton underwear, and replacing pantyhose with stockings and garters.

A yeast infection during pregnancy can be treated with over-the-counter drugs, but it's necessary to notify your doctor and discuss treatment first. Yeast infections mostly occur late in pregnancy when constipation can intensify.

Constipation
To help prevent constipation during pregnancy avoid refined grains and sugar, and eat plenty of fiber. Fiber is necessary to keep constipation in check. Fresh vegetables and fruit are good sources of fiber and contain important vitamins and minerals.* However, grains work the best to encourage elimination. Whole wheat bread (watch out for added rye and vinegar), and cereals that contain the maximum amount of bran provide good fiber. Oat bran is another very good source and can be sprinkled on hot or cold cereals, added to cottage cheese or cooked in various dishes. It's necessary to drink an adequate amount of water after eating a meal prepared with bran or other high fiber ingredients.

179

Another way to prevent constipation is to take a supplement such as Fibercon (if tolerated) with a full glass of water after a meal. The fiber in this supplement will help to soften the food just eaten. However, because fiber can interfere with vitamin absorption it's necessary to take vitamin supplements at least one hour before taking a fiber supplement.

Avoid commercial canned or fresh pears treated with pesticides because they retain pesticide residue more than other fruits.

Acid Reflux and Heartburn
Some experts suggest that eating a small amount of fatty food 30 minutes before a meal can help to reduce stomach acid and aid digestion. A doctor may recommend an over-the-counter medication. Tums is considered safe and may work best for the IC patient who experiences bladder pain with other acid-reduction medications. It is necessary to consult your doctor before taking over-the-counter medications.

Nausea
According to some experts women who get adequate vitamin B-6 and complex carbohydrates (whole, unrefined grains), and avoid a diet too high in protein may reduce nausea during pregnancy. However B-6 supplements are usually a bladder irritant for IC patients, so patients may want to get their B-6 from foods such as whole grains and fish (be sure to buy fish from a known source).

Migraines
Hormones may cause migraine headaches during pregnancy. Hormonal sensitivity is very individual, but the IC patient who experiences hormone related migraines with her menstrual cycle may react to the same hormones during her pregnancy. However, the IC patient may instead experience relief without the

"ups and downs" of her monthly cycle, or at least find improvement after the first trimester when progesterone levels drop and estrogen levels rise. Again, it is necessary to keep your doctor informed of problems, especially if you are accustomed to taking medications for your migraines.

Delivery and IC

IC patients don't usually experience a worsening of bladder symptoms during delivery, even though the bladder is affected during the different types of delivery. However, IC patients should plan and be prepared to deal with IC symptoms that could occur with, and/or after delivery. Researching and networking with other IC patients are very important. Refer to the *Interstitial Cystitis Survival Guide* by Robert M. Moldwin, M.D. for more information about delivery.

C-Section Delivery

When the IC patient has a C-section there's anesthesia and other medications to consider. There are decisions to make about being catheterized, as well as bladder-care after surgery. Networking with other IC patients who have had a C-section delivery will help. Working closely with your doctor and hospital staff is also necessary. *See Surgeries and Hospital Stays, Chapter Five.*

Vaginal Delivery

There are different factors to consider with a vaginal delivery. Although the IC patient may not have to worry about the medications needed during a C-section, she must consider how she will deal with her bladder during labor, an episiotomy (an incision made to increase the size of the vagina), and how she feels after delivery.

IC patients often need to pace and empty their bladders frequently to reduce the pain and pressure of bladder symptoms. Although a catheter may help some patients during labor, it may be an irritant to others or a limitation to those who must move around. Other considerations with a vaginal delivery include the possibility of needing repeated pelvic exams, drugs to induce labor, and of course, pain medication.

IC Pain after Pregnancy

Pelvic floor pain and spasms may occur after delivery, but IC patients often enjoy the lasting effects of estrogen after childbirth. The benefits of estrogen can last anywhere from six weeks to a few months. Patients who breast feed may not experience IC symptoms, migraines, or FMS until they finish breast feeding their babies.

Patients who do not breast feed can get back on their medications. Although not considered a standard treatment, some doctors suggest that women with IC or migraine symptoms may be helped by using an estradiol patch or topical gel until hormones are balanced. Other experts suggest that because progesterone levels are so high during pregnancy, mothers may be helped by taking natural progesterone to fight postpartum symptoms after they have delivered. Progesterone is not always tolerated by IC patients.

Some women have their first experience of IC symptoms after giving birth. Many different reasons have been speculated, such as hormonal changes and surgery when women have had a C-section. Because IC can be so unpredictable, IC patients should plan to have assistance with their babies until their symptoms are back in check.

Episiotomy

An antispasmodic, pain medication, an ice pack, and sometimes a catheter can be used to reduce inflammation, swelling, and pelvic floor spasms after an episiotomy. Warm baths are also helpful to soothe and aid the healing process. However, it's necessary to first ask the doctor if a bath is okay.

Caesarean Postpartum

As with other surgeries a patient must have time to recover. The IC patient may need IC treatments and extra help with her new lifestyle. She also may need to work closely with the doctor and/or a dietitian to get the needed nutrition to rebuild her body and take care of her new baby after surgery.

Breast Feeding

When breast feeding, women must continue with good nutritional habits. Breast feeding requires equal, if not more good nutrition than pregnancy. Although breast feeding is beneficial to a baby, new mothers with IC may need to get back on a diet for IC or take medication to control IC symptoms. Some mothers try to give their babies a little breast milk before switching to a bottle formula.

Breast feeding requires a woman to do with less sleep. Experts suggest that the new mother with IC express her milk so another person can feed the baby while mom gets some sleep.

Coping With a Newborn

It takes a lot of energy to cope with a newborn. The lack of sleep, occasional postpartum depression, the possibility of IC symptoms returning, the lifting, holding, and bending, plus the partner and other children in need of your attention can make life difficult. Planning for all of these factors and how to take care of yourself will help.

A massage after delivery may help relieve the physical changes your body has endured with pregnancy and delivery. Rearranging the physical environment in your home to suit your needs will also help. Asking for help from family and friends, and taking enough time to get back to a normal pace is necessary. Comparing yourself to other new mothers without IC should be avoided.

If there is any doubt that you are not physically and/or emotionally recovering from childbirth, you should ask to be tested for anemia and hypothyroidism. Pain and fatigue should not be taken for granted. IC experts recommend that a patient not wait until her first postpartum appointment to deal with concerns.

RESOURSES

Johnathan Bernstein, M.D.
Cincinnati, Ohio
(513) 931-0775

Slippery Stuff
1-800-759-7883

Harvard Women's Health Watch
P.O. Box 420234
Palm Coast, FL 32142-0234
1-800-829-5921
(Canadian subscribers) (904) 445-4662

There are new books addressing pregnancy for women with chronic conditions. There is also ongoing information for IC patients and pregnancy. *Contact the ICA, the IC Network, and other IC patients.*

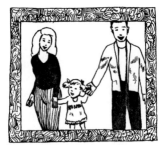

Chapter 9

LIVING WITH IC:
A SPOUSE'S PERSPECTIVE

Twelve years ago, when I first began dating my wife, I did not know much about IC, a chronic disease that has changed both our lives. I did know she was often in pain and had frequent urination. It was obvious that something was wrong. But like many people, I had little awareness of IC. Like most men, I had limited understanding of how problems can affect womens' bodies.

Then I began learning more and going with my wife to see the doctor. I was at her side when the diagnosis of IC was confirmed. As we grew closer and began building a life together, I have learned a great deal about IC. I now accept that this disease is part of my life, it is not going to go away and, most importantly, I have ways to deal with it.

I am also a psychologist. I directed a unit for patients who have Alzheimer's Disease which involved leading support groups for families of people with this chronic disease. Some might say that my professional training would make it easier for me to cope with a wife who has IC. From an objective point of view, it is true that I know a great deal about clinical ways to help families deal with disease.

Yet, because this disease is affecting me and my wife, I have many subjective feelings that are hard to ignore. Giving advice to others is much easier than incorporating that advice into my own life. This makes me just like other family members of IC patients. Even after living with IC for years, I do not always handle my feelings in constructive ways. I get angry, feel sorry for myself and feel sad.

At times I have felt resentful about vacations and special dinners that had to be canceled. Like many partners of IC patients, I have had to change my expectations about what life with my wife should be like. I have even perceived my wife as a bladder and forgotten she has other aspects to her identity.

IC is not just a physical disease. It has powerful emotional side effects, and it changes the way a family must live day-to-day. IC can interfere with everything from one's sex life to a party invitation from the boss, to the weekly trip to the grocery store. But, because most IC sufferers look healthy and are often young, it is difficult for significant others to accept the seriousness of the condition.

After dealing personally with all of these issues for many years, I have learned many ways to make life with an IC patient not only manageable, but also satisfying and rewarding in all the ways that we all want our marriages and families to be satisfying and rewarding. This is what I would like to tell other spouses and family members coping with IC.

Families need help and support because this disease will require great sacrifice and change. Spouses can run away or get trapped in denial, or they can go too far in the other direction and get so involved in taking care of their wives, they forget their own needs--even their own identities. Caregivers often need care as much as the patients.

There are many helpful tips I can offer to other families. Life with an IC patient will be easier, for example, if you avoid rush hour traffic and plan ahead by knowing where bathrooms are wherever you go. But rather than plunging in with advice, I think it is more helpful to look at the coping process more broadly, in a developmental and family context, so that the ways to live more reasonably with IC are considered in proper perspective.

What do I mean? Family members, just like the IC patient, will go through different stages of dealing with the disease, depending on their age, their situation, their awareness of what is actually happening with the patient, and her/his particular needs.

Everything will change, and continue to change. Even if you or others in your family are coping well with IC, this may change as you enter new phases of your life or deal with stressful situations. The birth of a baby, the IC patient's inability to continue working, cancellation of an anticipated family vacation, or when children reach adolescence--all can spark new stress. Stressful times do not always involve major life changes. For example, when the IC patient starts following the recommended diet, the relationship will be pressured. You may have to give up favorite foods and restaurants.

Once family members learn to accept and expect change, they'll be able to cope and adapt better, no matter how much their lives are altered. I like to think of living with an IC patient as a marathon, not a sprint. IC, as a chronic illness, is something family members and the patient will have to deal with over time.

Look at the contrast of a chronic illness such as IC with an acute illness like the flu. When a child has the flu, for instance, family members must make changes in their lives--call the doctor, stay home from work, get prescriptions filled, make chicken soup. But in a few days the child is well, and everyone returns to their normal routine. With IC, family members will have to continually make adjustments, year-after-year.

Learning to Accept IC

Given the constantly changing dynamics of the family, the most important thing families of IC patients can do is accept the disease and accept that it will continue to change their lives over time. Acceptance can be complex, and it does not happen overnight. In most cases IC comes on gradually, and patients will probably have symptoms for a long time before they are diagnosed and treated. In many cases, a patient and family will have been dealing with heavy-duty stress long before IC is diagnosed. You can expect the acceptance process to be quite different for the patient and family members. The IC patient may feel relieved at finally getting a diagnosis for her symptoms and knowing treatment is available. At the same time, family members may feel more confusion than relief.

IC may differ from other chronic diseases that have no cure, but it also is similar. In dealing with such diseases, denial always comes before acceptance. Most every family member, I believe, should expect to experience some denial about the reality and implications of IC. It may be useful to view this denial as the first stage of acceptance.

I have learned many ways to ease the acceptance process along. The most helpful thing is learning as much as possible about IC. I recommend accompanying your spouse to the doctor. This accomplishes several things. By listening to the doctor, you can better understand what your spouse is going through. You will get an opportunity to gain information about IC, ask questions and help your spouse remember the doctor's instructions.

And, just by being present, you are supporting your spouse. Sometimes doctors do not take the symptoms of IC patients seriously, so your presence is a powerful confirmation that your spouse is indeed suffering. Far too many doctors and nurses are uneducated about IC, so you, as a family member, will need to be an advocate for the patient. IC patients also get complacent. They hesitate to seek treatment. Going with your spouse helps her or him avoid passivity.

Learning as much as possible is crucial when dealing with IC. In some strange way, patients and family members would find it easier to deal with a more dangerous disease like cancer simply because it is better accepted and brings sympathy and compassionate responses from others. IC is not well-known, and because men do not understand the way the symptoms present themselves in the female body, it is easy to think that the patient should be able to control them. At some level, most of us fall into the trap of believing that people with urinary problems should be able to use willpower to control their symptoms.

There is nothing scarier than the unknown. With IC, the more you know the easier things will be. Being present and eager to learn can also put you in touch with encouraging news. I remember feeling comforted when the doctor told us that IC does not have to get worse with age.

Taking Control

Families of IC patients can cope better by gaining as much control as possible over their environment. One major way to take control is to plan ahead. Make planning in advance a way of life in every possible situation. There are many ways to accomplish this.

- Find bathrooms in advance. We know where every bathroom is located in the cities in which we have lived. While IC is not a psychosomatic disease, IC sufferers, like everyone else, are more likely to need to use the bathroom when they are anxious. Locating bathrooms eases anxiety on many levels.

- Learn to be flexible and give up strict time schedules. With practice, you can learn to allot more time than you will probably need for every activity. Always have a back-up plan ready.

- Schedule trips or special events when there is a good chance that the IC patient will feel strong. Many women with IC have symptoms that get worse according to their menstrual cycle. Do not plan events when symptoms are most severe.

- A major way IC sufferers can take control of their own lives is by following the recommended diet which my wife discusses in other chapters. The diet truly lessens frequency and pain of symptoms for most patients. But it is restrictive, so a spouse can be extremely supportive just by helping the patient stick with it. This was tough for me because I have been told that I do not eat to live, I live to eat. I love to eat out, so I did not like ruling out restaurants that do not serve what my wife can eat. We no longer go to French restaurants or share a bottle of wine over dinner. But because I accept that the diet is important and that my wife needs my support, these sacrifices are easier to make. When my wife feels better, I feel better. Now I know everything about my wife's diet. I read labels carefully. We work together as a team to help her stay on the diet. Working as a team will help both you and your spouse feel more in control and avoid stress.

Dealing with Feelings

I have felt the gamut of emotions since my wife began suffering from IC. What is particularly confounding about IC is that it stirs up so many conflicting feelings.

For example, I love my wife and want to help her feel healthy and feel good about herself, but no matter what I do, she still is in pain and still has to go to the bathroom all the time. I feel as if everything I try to do is useless. So I feel helpless, then angry, then guilty for feeling angry. This cycle of feelings will be all-too-familiar to family members of IC patients. I think that it is important to reassure IC patients and family members that these emotions are natural and normal. A spouse who feels such conflict is not a bad person.

The best way to deal with intense feelings is to acknowledge they exist and deal with them constructively. It does not help to try to cover them up or keep them inside until they come out in inappropriate ways, such as kicking a door. Good communications among family members is essential to this process.

Overall, I have dealt with negative feelings by learning to be realistic, especially about my expectations. I do not build up high hopes about anything. Then, when things do work out, I am pleasantly surprised. I have learned to be more realistic by increasing my knowledge of IC and giving myself some time. I have adjusted my thinking and my expectations for our lives together. In the process, my anger has gone away.

Early on, it is so important to alter your expectations of your partnership and your life, together and separately. I used to envision us taking vacations together, enjoying delicious dinners out and going to parties and special events. I have had to realize that my wife will not always feel well enough to be by my side. And, I have accepted the even harder reality that she may have to cancel plans at the last minute. Changing my expectations has helped me deal with my anger and frustration.

Let me point out that changing expectations does not guarantee that you will never feel angry again. I feel like I have come a long way in accepting my wife's IC, but I still get angry at her. When we have plans to go on a trip, I accept that it may have to be canceled, but I sometimes get mad if it happens.

Never compare persons with IC to other healthy persons. Not only is this unfair, it will increase frustrations. In many cases, it is not realistic to expect persons with IC to work. It is also not realistic for a patient's spouse to get his hopes up for sex on a certain night.

I remember getting angry soon after my wife was diagnosed because I had to buy the groceries. My wife was in too much pain to go to the store. Now I look at the situation more realistically and understand that she does not often feel well enough to shop. I was able to change my expectations and grocery shopping is not as burdensome.

I am a firm believer that counseling can be valuable to families living with IC. Talking with a professional can give you an objective look at ways you can de-stress your life, take control of the things you can and handle your negative feelings. My wife and I went to a social worker together and our lives are better as a result. We learned how to handle our negative feelings more effectively. For example, we made the joint decision to pay someone to do our laundry rather than getting upset over how and when it got done.

Family Dynamics

In my experience, dealing with IC caused my wife and me to take on distinct roles in the relationship. I began to see myself as the caregiver and my wife as the patient--or even worse, as a bladder. Of course, I am more than a caregiver, and my wife is more than a patient, even though we often assume those roles.

It is emotionally dangerous for family members of IC patients to define themselves in such rigid ways. I am more than a caregiver. I am a professional in the field of geriatrics. I am a friend to many people. I have outside interests other than IC. I have had to learn that I can still have a good day on a weekend when my wife is sick in bed. I can go out and enjoy myself without her. Luckily for me, my wife encourages me to do this.

It works the other way, too. Family members need to help the IC patient see her or his role as more than the "sick person" or victim. My wife has many interests, talents and dimensions. She is a whole person.

Both the IC patient and spouse must find ways to exercise their independence of the other at times and remember they are separate people with unique interests. This is something I continually work on in my life. It is easy for couples dealing with a chronic disease to become too intertwined in each other. This results in major problems. With an IC patient who has no children, the partner may fall even more easily into a caregiver role. Some spouses are so immersed in caring for their partners that they do not take care of themselves and their own needs.

At the other extreme, some men whose wives have IC run away. When an IC patient gets divorced, I suspect that the disease was not the only problem. In many cases, the couple may have had communication problems and other difficulties that IC brought to the surface.

Even when a couple has a solid relationship, they are constantly under stress because the spouse or partner of an IC patient must carry a heavier load in the marriage. And, IC also can cause financial problems if the patient can no longer work. The spouse or partner may have to take more responsibility for household management, errands, chores, and child-rearing. Good communication, making sure one's needs are met and recognizing your identity as a person separate from the disease and caregiving role are essential in alleviating such stress.

In the extended family of an IC patient, expect to encounter misunderstanding and denial, even from mothers and mother-in-laws whom you might think would be compassionate. Even family members who accept the disease will do so at different stages. It can be helpful to bring these family members to a support group meeting.

Giving family members time also helps. After a while, people do understand. Family gatherings can be a challenge, especially on holidays and special occasions when the IC patient's absence, pain or diet may become hot-button issues. Adjusting your own expectations and constant education of all family members can help.

How families with children can best deal with IC depends on many factors: ages of the children, how long a parent has suffered with IC and how well a family communicates and handles emotions. Working to maintain a good relationship is extremely important if a couple has children when IC is diagnosed. In these situations, the spouse or partner may feel overwhelmed with responsibility. Children need complete and total understanding, and a parent with IC will find supplying these qualities difficult at times.

Whatever the case in a particular family, children must always be told that their parent is sick so that they do not develop false expectations or misunderstanding. You can not hide the illness anyway, because even small children will be aware that something is wrong. They need to know that there will be times when their mother, or father, needs peace and quiet and may not be available to them. Young children can be extremely helpful when a parent is experiencing symptoms. They seem to have a sympathetic understanding. However, the same child may react quite differently upon reaching adolescence.

Children do have higher expectations than adults. So when planning with children, it helps to concentrate on brief high-quality activities and outings that the IC patient can handle. Even with IC, you can still be a good mother or father and make your children feel loved and secure.

Improving Communication

As I think about ways to cope with the presence of IC in a family and keep stress down and a marriage strong, I continually come back to the importance of good communication. Keeping communication open and effective is a basic strategy helpful in solving every problem that comes up when dealing with IC.

Good relationships are possible only when both parties tell each other what their needs are and feel that these needs are being met. They can not do this without good communication, which can be a challenge even under the best of circumstances. I mentioned the importance of counseling earlier. Another reason I recommend it is because it can improve communication and help couples see the bigger picture of their lives and relationship.

Good communication needs to be top-priority within a marriage, and outside of it, too. Everyone has to have someone other than their spouse to talk with. This is usually more difficult for men than for women. I speak from experience. Discussing my wife's illness is not what I want to do with other men while drinking a beer and watching a ball game. Fortunately, I happen to work with nurses, who are very supportive and helpful to me.

My wife learned early in her illness how vital it is for IC patients to find a good support group. I define a "good" support group as one which emphasizes positive coping and mutual help rather than pity. Encourage your spouse to find such a support group, and go with her occasionally. Talking with other people in the same situation can be invaluable. I am sorry to report there are not many support groups for the families of IC patients. Perhaps you can form your own.

Dealing with Other People

One of the many challenges of living with IC is coping with the reactions of other people. I can not say this enough: IC is not easily understood. How do you explain needing time off from work to go to a doctor's appointment? How do you respond when new friends invite you and your wife to a party?

I feel it is best to tell friends and family members the truth about IC. Being truthful does not mean telling everyone everything or expecting them to completely understand. You can decide in advance how much is appropriate to reveal in certain situations. I have told my employers that my wife has a chronic bladder disease, and I often receive supportive, positive responses.

It has also helped my wife and me to stay on the same social program. We keep our expectations of our social life toned down and decide together what we are going to do. Even so, going to parties and the homes of friends is hard. If we accept an invitation, we have to somehow tell the hosts that my wife has a chronic disease and can only eat certain foods. This can be tough. I remind myself that friends who do not understand are not really good friends.

I said earlier that living with IC in a family is like running a marathon. To take this analogy further, the only way to run a marathon successfully, or live with IC successfully, is to learn new skills, stretch your abilities and put in a lot of practice. Having many strategies available to address problems is important. The support of other people cheering you on is essential. In sharing my experiences living with IC, I hope to send you off on your own successful marathon of living more happily, despite the presence of this chronic disease.

Chapter 10
COLLECTING & SHARING INDIVIDUAL STORIES

Bert: Teen Struggles Alone

Bert's first episode of IC occurred at the age of 17 after her first sexual encounter. She had used a diaphragm which resulted in a bladder infection. The antibiotic she was prescribed did not work and made her bladder symptoms worse. Although the second antibiotic she was given cleared up her infection, Bert continued to experience bladder pain. Her unexplained pain was treated with a low dose antibiotic, Pyridium, and bladder instillations made of olive oil and camphor for six years.

When Bert was 22 she had laser surgery for papillomavirus. After the surgery she had problems with yeast and an increase in bladder pain. She also began to experience vulvar vestibulitis. Her urologist treated her with DMSO instillations which were extremely painful. Bert discontinued DMSO treatment when she found she was given treatment while having a bladder infection.

Determined to find the cause of, and treatment for her bladder pain, Bert had two cystoscopies within six months. After the second cystoscopy she was diagnosed with IC and referred to a neurosurgeon for back surgery to correct her bladder symptoms. Back surgery did not correct Bert's bladder symptoms. Several months after her surgery Bert returned to the same urologist for another surgery. During this surgery the urologist removed infected nerve ganglia via laparoscopy which successfully relieved her vulvar vestibulitis, but also triggered her IC symptoms.

Bert began to experience back problems about a year after her surgeries. Her new back pain interfered with her career as a graphic designer. Bert found that she had to give up her exercise routine of running. When she tried to reach the doctor who performed her back surgery, he would not return her calls. She saw a neurologist, who could not help. She tried acupuncture, sports medicine and myofascial therapy. Although none of these therapies stabilized her back pain, the myotherapy seemed to give her some relief. However, she now needed to take Ativan to relieve her back pain. Sitting all day at work was becoming impossible. Still in her 20's, Bert came to terms with her situation. Realizing that her early experience with pain, doctors and therapists had given her a special understanding of the emotional effects of a chronic disease, Bert made the choice to change her career and help others as a therapist in the mental health field.

Bert's new life brought some very good changes. She found a doctor who treated her symptoms with doxepin which helped her vulvar vestibulitis, bladder and back pain. She began to eliminate foods high in oxalates to control her vulvar vestibulitis. She also eliminated foods high in acid to control her IC. And, she finally found a way to control her yeast problem without vaginal creams, by using boric acid capsules and oral fluconazole (Diflucan). However, her health problems were not all under control. Bert began to experience anxiety, weight gain and exhaustion. She was diagnosed with hypothyroidism, and after a trial period on synthetic thyroid medication, Bert switched to natural thyroid which she found more agreeable. Bert also began taking Benadryl to treat allergic reactions and sinus pain. Bert soon learned to live her life at a slower pace and managed to continue with her art work on the side.

Due to her recent education, career change and slower lifestyle, Bert has a new perspective. During one of her first job interviews in the mental health field she was told that she was too young and inexperienced to understand the depth of a patient's problems. Bert remembers thinking: "I look healthy, young and possibly as though I haven't experienced much pain in my own life. However, I have endured several painful, invasive, unproductive medical procedures in my twenties, and I have a long history of dealing mostly on my own with a little recognized illness. My identity has been confusing and I sometimes become frustrated with myself because I can't seem to do what other peers seem able to do."

Bert has achieved more in her lifetime than most women in their early 30's. She leads a full and productive life and does not intend to limit herself until she must.

Elizabeth: Relief in Pregnancy

Elizabeth is an active mother of two in her late 30's. Her problems began with repeated bladder infections during her early 20's. Her infections were treated with antibiotics. When her infections finally subsided she continued to experience bladder pain for a year or so. Although Elizabeth eventually felt better she starting having intermittent episodes of deep vaginal burning with vague bladder pain. Elizabeth also found intercourse painful. The doctors she saw diagnosed her with yeast or vaginal infections, but treatment did not help or change her intermittent pain.

Elizabeth's problems were soon compounded with chest wall pain which was misdiagnosed as pleurisy. Elizabeth also began to suffer with terrible back pain due to a ruptured disc, but she was misdiagnosed and told she had a sprained back. Elizabeth tried many different therapies to treat her back pain, including chiropractic adjustments, physical therapy, myofascial release, and acupuncture, but she found no relief. During her search for pain management, the pain from her ruptured disc spread from her lower to her upper back, neck and jaw.

Elizabeth continued to fight her pain. She was now in her 30's and healthcare professionals were telling her to see a therapist. She was told that her untreatable pain was probably due to too much stress, unresolved childhood issues or other emotional problems. Elizabeth saw a therapist for two years, but therapy did not help her pain at all. She went back to treating her physical symptoms. She was treated with appliances for TMJ (temporomandibular joint) disorder. She also tried Craniosacral treatment. When the practitioners at the TMJ clinic saw no improvement in Elizabeth's pain they referred her back to the orthopedic doctor who now properly diagnosed her with a ruptured disk. Elizabeth then tried more physical therapy, as well as other therapies, but nothing helped her general muscle pain and her bladder pain was now almost unbearable.

At 33, Elizabeth was diagnosed with IC (her brother was diagnosed with IC a few years later). The hydrodistention used during the cystoscopy helped alleviate her symptoms for at least six months. When she returned to her urologist for help he gave her another cystoscope to verify her diagnosis of IC. This time the procedure made her symptoms much worse. Elizabeth tried DMSO, but could not tolerate it. She took amitriptyline which didn't help. During this time she also tried other drugs, such as Flexeril, to treat her muscle pain, but these drugs set off her bladder pain. She was diagnosed with fibromyalgia and prescribed nortriptyline and Klonopin. Both helped her muscle pain without triggering her IC. Elizabeth then followed a diet for IC and continued to try different drugs to control her bladder pain. Elizabeth did not experience frequency with her IC.

When Elizabeth was in her mid-30's she and her husband tried to get pregnant. Elizabeth underwent fertility treatment which did work. Pregnancy helped everything. The muscle and bladder pain were gone. She didn't need her drugs, however, she stayed on a restricted diet for IC and was afraid to take prenatal vitamins. In her third trimester Elizabeth found that she could eat almost everything except acidic foods. Three months after her little boy was born her bladder and muscle pain returned. Elizabeth tried exercise and a mind/body program which she found detrimental to her IC. Although she had no trouble following the breathing and pain awareness exercises, they increased her pain as she became more aware of it. The instructor told her to "just work through it." Elizabeth explained that IC patients must use distraction to deal with their bladder pain, but the instructor could not accept this fact. Frustrated, Elizabeth resumed the drugs she had previously taken.

Through fertility treatments, which aggravated her IC, Elizabeth became pregnant again. During the time of these treatments the doctors found some endometriosis, however, pregnancy improved everything and made her bladder pain go away. Elizabeth ate fruit and took prenatal vitamins. She still had some muscle pain (which she tried treating with neuromuscular therapy) and she experienced a little incontinence during the latter part of pregnancy and postpartum. Kegel exercises prescribed for incontinence did not help, but the incontinence eventually went away on its own. Like her first pregnancy, Elizabeth's IC pain returned exactly three months after her baby girl's birth. This time, though, the pain was worse.

Elizabeth quit her demanding full-time position and began working as a part-time consultant. She also began taking Elmiron. Raising children can be difficult for Elizabeth when she is experiencing pain, but her children have also been a wonderful distraction. For the most part they are Elizabeth's salvation.

Elizabeth continues to look for relief and a drug that will last. Elmiron quit helping after nine months so she discontinued it. Elizabeth, in need of relief, is now giving the Elmiron another try for at least three months. She is taking it along with tricyclic antidepressants this time. However, she is wondering if the Elmiron is causing her irritable bowel syndrome to act up, because she is now experiencing diarrhea. Elizabeth is considering having an epidural if these drugs do not help her IC pain.

Elizabeth also suffers with allergies, asthma and osteoarthritis in her spine, but she places treatment for her bladder pain first. With her diligence, willpower and determination, as well as her love for her family, Elizabeth will probably find the relief she has been seeking for years.

Peggy: Tale of a Survivor

Peggy, like many other IC patients, experienced urinary frequency as a child. When Peggy reached her 20's she began to suffer with bladder infections, which were repeatedly treated with antibiotics. When Peggy was in her early 30's, she began experiencing irregular menstrual bleeding and colon problems. Peggy was diagnosed with endometriosis and underwent four D & C procedures (dilatation and curettage) as treatment. At the age of 37, Peggy was prescribed diuretics for high blood pressure. Soon after beginning her new medication she began experiencing severe bladder pain and frequency. The urologist she saw treated her with urethral dilations and Peggy somehow managed to get on with her work which involved traveling. When Peggy was 39 she was told that she was officially in menopause which explained her earlier symptoms of irregular bleeding and colon problems. However, when Peggy was prescribed opposed estrogen (with progestin) her bladder symptoms flared-up. Thinking the pain and frequency was caused by a bladder infection, Peggy got a prescription for antibiotics. The antibiotics exasperated her bladder pain, but no doctor could explain her symptoms. Four painful years later, Peggy was diagnosed with interstitial cystitis.

Peggy read as much as possible and attended a support group to learn more about IC. She discontinued opposed estrogen and began taking unopposed estrogen. Her bladder symptoms soon improved. She found further relief having DMSO treatments and following a diet for IC. However, Peggy's health problems continued in a rapid domino effect. Not long after her diagnosis of IC, she was diagnosed with irritable bowel syndrome, hypothyroidism and pernicious anemia. Peggy also began to experience menstrual bleeding, but the unopposed estrogen kept her bladder symptoms calm, so she continued to take it. When the bleeding became serious, Peggy was admitted to the hospital for an emergency hysterectomy to stop precancerous hyperdysplasia. During her hysterectomy Peggy also received manipulation to free a frozen shoulder that had been unsuccessfully treated until this time.

After recovering from the hysterectomy, Peggy experienced a certain amount of relief, but she started having problems with one of her eyes. A doctor diagnosed her with glaucoma, and then found an arachnoid (brain cyst) on an MRI which was putting pressure on her optic nerve. After this upsetting news Peggy had a two year grace period with no unusual problems.

When Peggy experienced chest pain she didn't think much of it. Peggy knew that other IC patients experienced chest pain. However, when the pain became severe she knew she had to see her doctor. Once again, Peggy was admitted for surgery. This time she had her gall bladder removed.

Peggy now considers herself a survivor of the surgeries and the side effects of different medications. When asked how she has coped, Peggy explains, "I have found that to cope with IC is an 'everyday' experience because each day is different. There are some very good days and some very bad days. This condition is chronic and constant. Diet and anxiety play a large role in how my IC is affecting me, but I can never really pinpoint what has set off a pain pattern. I do know that walking for a period of time (more than a half an hour) will set off a terrible pain spasm that will put me in bed for several days. Rest, with my legs elevated will ease the pain. Also, unopposed estrogen has done wonders for my well-being. My IC symptoms are more manageable while taking estrogen. My doctors cannot explain why, but I know that estrogen helps to make me feel better."

Peggy now lives in a small city and so far she has only found a few understanding doctors. She can no longer get DMSO treatments or much compassion for her IC, but she is somehow managing well. Peggy stays in touch with the friends she made through an IC support group. These friends think that Peggy is more of a survivor than she will ever know.

Gillian: Coping with Overlapping Conditions
Health problems occurred throughout Gillian's life. At age 11 she repeated a school year because of a systemic strep infection. In high school she was diagnosed as borderline diabetic. She often hid the fatigue she felt. When she went away to college Gillian physically fell apart, and dropped out after eight weeks of dormitory life and early classes. The doctors she saw could not find the problem, although she complained of feeling like she had mononucleosis. With rest she could barely manage, but she could not hold down a job without becoming exhausted. The more tired she became the less she could sleep, and at least every three weeks she would go to bed with flu-like symptoms and a bad sore throat. Her doctors referred her to a psychiatrist who prescribed sleeping pills and tranquilizers which made her feel worse. Gillian became afraid and began to hide her illness when she realized that no doctor or person in her life could really understand, except for her mother who had fought polio and glandular fever, or what is now sometimes considered chronic fatigue syndrome. Desperate for relief, Gillian moved to a city known for its alternative lifestyles to learn about holistic medicine.

Gillian improved after her move and learned how to cope with her bouts of flu symptoms, as well as a new symptom, urinary frequency. However, six years later after another move, Gillian woke up one morning with terrible vaginal pain which sent her to the floor. The gynecologist found nothing and fortunately, the pain did not return though Gillian began to suffer with sinus infections. She gave up dairy products which seemed to help. Four years after her first episode with allergies Gillian began to experience a spastic colon whenever she had her familiar flu symptoms, about every three weeks. A year or so later Gillian began to suffer with muscle stiffness and pain in her left lower back, in the front of her hips and in her feet. The new symptoms intensified in late ovulation. A doctor prescribed nystatin to treat yeast. The awful vaginal pain she had experienced years ago returned and was now accompanied with unbearable urinary frequency. She was given antibiotics for a bladder infection. Her discomfort, pain and frequency worsened. She saw a new gynecologist who told her she had interstitial cystitis and referred her to a urologist who would not perform a cystoscopy, but advised her to follow Dr. Larrian Gillespie's IC diet. The diet helped for about nine months, but Gillian eventually became very ill and her terrible bladder and vaginal pain became chronic. She saw a new gynecologist who took her to the urologist's office across the hall. A cystoscope diagnosed her with IC. After the cystoscopy Gillian experienced heavy bleeding, but her IC symptoms gradually improved, for awhile.

Gillian's first oral treatment was an experimental drug for IC called Elmiron. The new drug helped her bladder symptoms, but she discontinued it because it affected her spastic colon and made her very nauseated. She continued to follow the diet, but Gillian became seriously ill about six months later when she broke out in severe hives, experienced swelling and a temporary paralysis in her arms. She was diagnosed with autoimmune arthritis caused by some allergic reaction. Although she got over her condition after taking steroids for four months, she never felt the same and continued to show red streaking on her skin. Gillian also showed high prolactin levels. Fortunately, an MRI showed no tumor on her pituitary gland. But, now her mid-cycle symptoms of pelvic, hip and leg pain became severe. Her IC pain was also intensifying so she began DMSO treatments which were very helpful.

Gillian's doctor performed a laparoscopy but found no signs of endometriosis. However, a sigmoidoscopy and induced menopause, with the injected drug Lupron, proved that her pain was due to colon spasms caused by hormonal changes. The induced menopause got rid of all of her muscle pain, stiffness and colon pain, but her bladder pain reared up after three months of injections. Gillian discontinued the Lupron, took temporary estrogen replacement and began taking amitriptyline, which helped her bladder and some of her colon problems. Nevertheless, Gillian's pelvic, hip and leg pain continued to grow worse during mid-month. She was diagnosed with fibromyalgia and a bulging fifth lumbar disc, as well as bursitis in her hips.

During these years of continuous health problems Gillian experienced severe reactions to all kinds of cleaning products, perfumes and paints. As her sensitivity became worse she felt heart palpitations, numbness and tingling in her hands, as well as slurred speech. She was diagnosed with mitral valve prolapse. Not long after her new diagnoses Gillian also started breaking out in bright red hives that felt and looked like bug bites. The hives eventually covered areas of her face, legs and arms. She was told she had psoriasis, but the sun and chemical fumes made it worse and it never went away. She was treated with the chemo drug methotrexate, but could not tolerate the IC symptoms it triggered in her bladder. Gillian also began to have trouble focusing her eyes. A neuro-opthamologist diagnosed her with fibromyalgia in the muscles of her eyes. Her next doctor visit would, however, be the most surprising.

During a routine exam with her general practitioner, Gillian's doctor discovered a lump on her thyroid. Gillian had two thyroid surgeries that showed both follicular and papillary thyroid cancer. Gillian was given an oral radioactive cocktail and was confined to isolation for four days in a room that was covered and padded in plastic diapers, clear plastic and tape.

Fortunately, the iodine and radioactive cocktail did not affect her bladder, except with frequency, but the room and the radiation made her feel very ill. Her oncologist told her to "suck it up" when she complained. Gillian's urologist, surgeon (who was her urologist's brother) and gynecologist were wonderful.

It has been four years since her cancer surgery and Gillian has been diagnosed with pernicious anemia and fibromyalgia which was confirmed with a new blood test. Gillian attributes the positive blood work for fibromyalgia to an early pool injury that resulted in two pieces of silicone embedded in her knee.

When Gillian looks back on her experiences she says that so much has happened she can't remember what she felt like in her healthier years. In hindsight, she rates the pain of IC as the worse thing she has dealt with. Equal to her bladder pain is her sadness that she has a disease which is experimented on animal models. And, although Gillian is very happy with some of her doctors, she ranks the challenges, difficulties, and misdiagnoses and judgment from different doctors and alternative healthcare practitioners as the next hardship.

Holly: Mid-life Diagnosis and Disability

Holly was diagnosed with interstitial cystitis at age 43. In retrospect, Holly recalls suffering with numerous bladder infections that went untreated as a child. Trips in the family car were difficult for her, as well as for her family members who blamed nervousness as the cause of Holly's urinary frequency. Looking back, Holly also remembers having a fear of sleeping over with friends. The bladder pain and frequency she experienced from undiagnosed urinary tract infections (UTIs) interfered with a normal childhood.

Holly was fairly symptom-free in her 20's and 30's, except for occasional urgency and frequency. She didn't think much of these symptoms because they had been normal for her since childhood. However, when Holly was 42 the pain she experienced during her childhood returned. Wondering if the pain was caused by a yeast infection, Holly began researching her symptoms. While looking through the book, *The New Our Bodies, Ourselves*, she discovered that her symptoms sounded a lot like those of interstitial cystitis. Under an extremely painful cystoscopy performed without anesthesia, Holly was diagnosed with IC. Not long after her diagnosis other uncomfortable symptoms started to flare-up. She began having problems with her colon and she began experiencing general muscle pain. At age 44 she was diagnosed with fibromyalgia.

Holly completely changed her lifestyle in order to cope with her different symptoms. Taking medication was almost impossible because she had many drug sensitivities. Holly found that if she laid down, or at least put her feet up halfway through the day, she could usually control the inflammation she experienced. However, when her IC pain reached a "ten", she needed to take Percocet. Yet, like many other IC patients, Holly found that even Percocet hardly relieved her IC pain. When Holly turned 46 she decided to have a laparoscopy to further investigate the cause of her pain.

Holly was diagnosed with endometriosis and treated with laser surgery. Although she did not experience much IC pain after the procedure, Holly did have extensive vaginal bleeding. And, although the procedure helped her pain, her periods became heavier and she began to suffer from iron deficient anemia. Holly tried many different iron supplements, but because of her irritable bowel syndrome and her IC she could not tolerate any supplement for long. Her doctor was concerned and had her try an IV iron drip, but she had a very severe reaction to it. Holly finally decided to add as much iron as possible to her diet to see her through menopause which she was told would help her improve her anemia.

Menopause brought on more symptoms which included heart palpitations. Holly knew that she had mitral valve prolapse, but she was still concerned. Her doctor thought it was

normal to experience an increase in palpitations during menopause, however, Holly began to experience more fatigue than
usual along with a deep feeling of depression. Holly decided to
have her thyroid level checked. Her blood work showed that
she had Hashimoto's thyroiditis, an autoimmune disease. Her
doctor was not surprised because he thought that her IC was an
autoimmune disease. When Holly learned that her newly diagnosed disease was hereditary she realized she shared the similar
problems of her mother and sister who both suffered with fibromyalgia.

It has now been six years after her diagnosis of IC and
other overlapping conditions. Holly can no longer work as a
full-time hairdresser. Physical exercise, including walking and
sitting for any length of time, is very difficult. Riding in certain
vehicles is often intolerable. Sexual activity results in extreme
pain for days after. With the help of a lawyer after two denials,
Holly now receives total disability for IC, which she feels is by
far her worst disease.

When Holly looks back she sums up her feelings, "Dealing with chronic conditions, especially IC, has been a lengthy
road of peaks and valleys. There is always some degree of pain,
but if my life remains calm with little stress, I can usually keep
my symptoms under control. However, most prescription
medications have contributed to my pain. I am very careful to
avoid drugs with many fillers and dyes because they cause such
razor blade pain in my bladder."

At times, Holly has risked her life to avoid the consequences of medications. However, sometimes Holly must take
a strong medication to control her pain. In her words, "If I were
to live a semblance of a normal and productive life, I would
need strong pain medication to just dull the pain, and that will
be my road less traveled if I can be helped by the rest."

Holly has a fighting spirit and has helped many IC patients as an activist for IC, presenting testimonials to state representatives for handicapped parking and "Potty Parity" rights for

IC patients. Holly is successfully recovering from a hysterectomy. Her gynecologist worked closely with her urologist during the surgery which involved the removal of two large fibroid cysts. Although Holly is now dealing with the side effects of the drugs used during and after her surgery, she does feel a sense of relief from the terrible pressure in her pelvic area.

Belle Judy: Early Days of IC

Growing up in the 40's and 50's, Belle Judy was considered "sickly." She suffered with bouts of flu, pernicious anemia and a serious kidney infection. In her late 20's she saw a specialist for arthritis in her hands and feet. She was diagnosed with arthritis which the doctor said was caused by kidney and bladder infections. He gave her a series of antibiotic shots. Belle Judy's arthritis did not go away. She decided to see a urologist. The urologist saw no signs of infection, but during a cystoscopy he found an inflamed patch which he said might feel like a blister in her bladder. Belle was given silver nitrate treatments. She felt no bladder symptoms before, during or after the treatments.

When Belle Judy was in her early 30's she began experiencing repeated yeast infections. A doctor removed her Bartholin's glands which have ducts that open into the vulva. After the surgery she experienced a pulling sensation in her urethra due to scarring. Urination didn't feel the same. When Belle approached menopause in her early 40's, she began to suffer with vulvar and urethral pain and swelling, as well as burning after urination. As menopause grew closer Belle began to experience pelvic pain, irritating bowel symptoms, and back and leg pain. She was diagnosed with IC, irritable bowel syndrome, fibromyalgia, osteoporosis, and arthritis in her lumbar spine and hip. She also displayed several symptoms of thyroid disease, but always tested within the normal range.

Belle eventually tried to treat her IC with DMSO treatments, but the treatments made her symptoms much worse. She tried taking Uristat, but it interfered with her irritable bowel management. Following a diet for IC also had a bad effect on her irritable bowel symptoms, because of the lack of fruit. Belle found she absolutely had to eat some fruit to manage. She did, however, need to eliminate caffeine and eat bland foods to control her IC symptoms.

When Belle tried estrogen replacement she experienced terrible migraine headaches and increased bladder pain. The estrogen also made her dizzy. Belle finally gave up on medications and hormone replacement. Instead she decided to follow a bland diet, to use ice to treat her pain and to live a restful, solitary life with very little exercise or walking.

Belle is now 61. Although she still suffers with a great deal of pain, she has made the courageous decision to venture out, travel, see the world, and live the rest of her life as fully as possible. So far, Belle has taken one fairly long trip which turned out to be more successful than she could have ever imagined. Belle is quite remarkable considering the world she endured before much was known about IC.

REFERENCES

American Medical Association. (1989). *Home medical encyclopedia.* New York: Random House.

Anstett, P. (Newspaper article) (1997). Bladder treatment shows promise. *Detroit Free Press, November 4.*

Antispasmodics: Anaspaz, Cystospas, Ditropan, Levsin, Levsinex, Urispas & Urised. (Internet website) (1996). *The IC Network.*

Aston, J., & Pollock, J. (1996). Aston-Patterning: Integrating Aston concepts into a massage therapy practice. *Massage, 60,* 30-35.

Benign cysts. (1999). *Harvard Women's Health Watch, August.*

Biofeedback shows promising results for IC and vulvar pain. (1994). *ICA Update. The Interstitial Cystitis Association, Spring.*

Bladder holding protocol. (Internet website) (1996). *The IC Network.*

Brooks, D. (1996). Boston panel on Fibromyalgia and CFS. *Massage Therapy Journal, Summer.*

Caudill, M.A. (1995). *Managing pain before it manages you.* New York: Guilford Press.

Chalker, R. (1997). Interstitial Cystitis. *Publication Of The American Foundation for Urologic Disease, Summer.*

Chalker, R., & Whitmore, K.E. (1990). *Overcoming bladder disorders.* New York:

Chinese herb study completed. (Internet website) (1997). *The Interstitial Cystitis Association. ICA Update, 3.*

Ciba-Geigy Corporation. (1995). *The menopause handbook.*

Curatek. (1996). *Bacterial Vaginosis. The most common vaginal infection.*

Domingue, G.J., & Ghoniem, G.M. (1997). Occult infection in Interstitial Cystitis. In G.R. Sant (Ed.). *Interstitial Cystitis* (pp. 77-86). Philadelphia: Lippincott-Raven.

Dreher, H. (1993). Proven mind/body medicine. *Natural Health, May/June.*

Enjoying intimacy in spite of the pain and fatigue. (1997). *Fibromyalgia Network, April.*

EPA tests fragranced products & indoor environments. (1991). *The Delicate Balance, 4,* 25-26.

Estrogen for heart disease: Risk or benefit? (2000). *Harvard Women's Health Watch, June.*

Estrogen update. (1999). *Harvard Women's Health Watch,* June.

FDA approves Elmiron, first oral treatment for IC. (1996). *The ICA Update. The Interstitial Cystitis Association, Fall.*

FDA approves natural progesterone. (1998). *Harvard Women's Health Watch, July.*

Federal court rules that IC is a disability. (1996). *The ICA Update. The Interstitial Cystitis Association, Fall.*

Fibromyalgia Syndrome and Chronic Fatigue Syndrome. (1996). *Fibromyalgia Network.* Tucson, AZ.

Folic acid fortification: Is it enough? (1998). *Harvard Women's Health Watch, February.*

Forecasting hot flashes. (1996). *Harvard Women's Health Watch, December.*

Gaby, A.R. (Reprint) (1997). Estrogen replacement therapy. *Women's Health Connection for Women's International Pharmacy, June.*

Getting estrogen through the skin. (1998). *Harvard Women's Health Watch, December.*

Gibson, B. (Handout). Interstitial Cystitis: The bladder infection that isn't. Suncoast GFIDS Support Group.

Gibson, B.A. (1995). *The Fibromyalgia handbook.* (2nd ed.). HarperCollins.

Gillespie, L. (1986). *You don't have to live with cystitis.* New York: Rawson Associates.

Gittes, R., & Nakamura, R. (Internet website) (1996). Female urethral syndrome: An infection of the female prostate glands? *The IC Network.*

Gorman, C. (1993). *Less toxic living* (6th ed.). Texarkana, Tx.

Hanno, P.M. (Ed.). (1994). *The urologic clinics of North America.* Philadelphia: W.B. Saunders.

Hect, M. (Newspaper article) (1998). Interstitial Cystitis is chronic and often hard to diagnose. *The Times-Picayune, June 24.*

Hohenfellner, M., Linn, J., Hampel, C., & Thuroff, J.W. (1997). Surgical treatment of Interstitial Cystitis. In G.R. Sant (Ed.). *Interstitial Cystitis* (pp. 223-233). Philadelphia: Lippincott-Raven.

How does FMS affect pregnancy? (1997). *Fibromyalgia Network, July.*

How estrogen works. (1998). *Harvard Women's Health Watch, April.*

How far will digestive problems go to disrupt your day? (1997). *Fibromyalgia Network, January.*

IC treatments. Alternative & holistic approaches. (Internet website) (1998). *Patient handbook. The IC Network.*

Inside Answers. (Webletter) *Insider. The Johns Hopkins Health, 1.*

Interstitial Cystitits: A bladder disorder (Internet website). *National Kidney and Urologic Disease Information Clearinghouse.*

Interstitial Cystitis. (1999). *National Institute of Diabetes and Digestive and Kidney Diseases, 99-3220.*

It's all about balance. *Women's health connection.* Complementary Issue III.

Jackson, N.D., & Teague, T. (1975). *The handbook for alternatives to chemical medicine.* Oakland, CA.

Kendall, J. (EPA study) (1991). Twenty most common chemicals found in thirty-one fragrance products. *Health Hazard Information. Citizens For A Toxic-Free Marin.*

Kengia, S. (Internet website) (2000). An interview with Dr. Stanley Jacob: Discussing DMSO. *DMSO.*

Koziol, J.A., Clark, D.C., Gittes, R.F., & Tan, E.M. (1993). The natural history of Interstitial Cystitis: A survey of 374 patients. *The Journal Of Urology, 149,* 465-469.

La Rock, D.R., & Sant, G.R. (1997). Intravesical therapies for Interstitial Cystitis. In G.R. Sant (Ed.). *Interstitial Cystitis* (pp. 247-255). Philadelphia: Lippincott-Raven.

Lack of noise filtering. Could it be causing your symptoms? (1996). *Fibromyalgia Network, April.*

Laumann, B. (1998). *A taste of the good life: A cookbook for an Interstitial Cystitis diet*. Tustin, CA: Freeman Family Trust Publications.

Low dose estrogen for bone loss. (1998). *Harvard Women's Health Watch, May*.

Low-dose estrogen for HRT. (1996). *Harvard Women's Health Watch, December*.

Markowitz, L. (1996). Minding the body, embodying the mind. *Networker, September/October*, 21-33.

McCormick, N., & Brookhoff, D. (1993). Perspective: Coping with IC. Managing chronic and severe bladder pain: Physicians and patients working together. *The Interstital Cystitis Association. ICA Update, 8*.

Medtronic announces FDA approval of Interstim therapy for urinary control. (Internet website) (1999). *Medtronic Press Release*.

Menopause: A new beginning. (Magazine) (1997). *Health And Fitness Magazine, September/October*.

Menzies, R. (1977). *The herbal dinner. A renaissance of cooking*. Millbrae, CA: Celestial Arts.

Merck Research Laboratories. (1997). *The Merck manual*. Whitehouse Station, N.J.: Merck & Co.

Messing, E.M., & Stamey, T.A. (1978). Interstitial Cystits. Early diagnosis, pathology and treatment. *Urology, 12,* 381-392.

Midlife menopause update. (1998). *Harvard Women's Health Watch, August.*

Mitral valve prolapse and medical testing. (1999). *Harvard Women's Health Watch, 7.*

Natural progesterone and synthetic progestins. *Women's health connection,* Complementary Issue II.

New approaches to PMS. (1998). *Harvard Women's Health Watch, February.*

New plant-based estrogen reduces osteoporosis risk. (Newspaper article) (1998). *The Times-Picayune.*

New standards for nutrients. (1998). *Harvard Women's Health Watch, June.*

New treatment for IC announced in Canada. (1995). *The ICA Update. The Interstitial Cystitis Association, Spring.*

Non-drug, hands-on and do-it-yourself therapies. (1996). *Fibromyalgia Network,October.*

Nutritional Supplements. (Internet website) (1996*). The Interstital Cystitis Network.*

O'Brien, T. (Newspaper article) (1998). Facts that figure into the stress picture. *The Times-Picayune,* February 5.

Parsons, C. L. (1993). Doctor's forum. *The Interstitial Cystitis Association. ICA Update, 8.*

Parsons, C.L. (1996). Doctor's forum. *The ICA Update. The Interstital Cystitis Association, Fall.*

Peters, K. (Internet website) (1999). ICN chat transcript. *Interstitial Cystitis Network, May 19.*

Pharmacist's guide to over-the counter and natural remedies. (1999). Rutherford, NJ: Avery Publishing.

Physicians desk reference. (1999). Montvale, NJ: Medical Economics Company.

Prelief study completed by Dr. Kristene Whitmore: Results are encouraging. (Internet website) *The Interstitial Cystitis Association.*

Potter, J. (1999). Tectonic changes in disability law. *Fibromyalgia Network, July.*

Progesterone. (1999). *Harvard Women's Health Watch, July.*

Research update: Connections between IC, Vulvodynia, and Fibromyalgia to be investigated. (1994). *The ICA Update. The Interstitial Cystitis Association, Summer.*

Sans Brochure. (Internet website) (1999). *Urosurge.*

Sant, G. (1994). Doctor's forum. *The ICA Update. The Interstitial Cystitis Association, Winter.*

Sant, G.R. (Ed.). (1997). *Interstitial Cystitis.* Philadelphia: Lippincott-Raven.

Scant evidence for progesterone cream. (1999). *Harvard Women's Health Watch, October.*

Self-help. (Pamphlet) (1992). *The Interstitial Cystitis Association.*

Simmons, K., & Norris, E. (1999). A test for Fibro? *Fibromyalgia Wellness Letter, 2, 4.*

Some suggested vulvar pain & itching measures. (Handout) (1993). *Adapted from the Vulvar Pain Foundation and the Interstitial Cystitis Association.*

Some tests you may not need. (1998). *Harvard Women's Health Watch, April.*

Stocker, C. (Newspaper article). (1994). Healthy houses. Indoor pollution can cause allergies and illnesses, but remedial measures are often simple. *The Boston Globe, December 8.*

Taking charge of Interstitial Cystitis. (1994). *Harvard Women's Health Watch, November.*

Tenenbaum, S.A, Rice, J.C., Espinoza, L.R., Cuellar, M.L. , Plymale, D.R., Sander, D.M., Willamson, L.L., Haislip, A.M., Gluck, O.S., Tesser, J.R., Nogy, L., Stribrny, K.M., Bevan, J.A., & Garry, R.F. (1997). Use of antipolymer antibody assay in recipients of silicone breast implants. *The Lancet. 349,* 449-454.

The inside story. A guide to indoor air quality. (1993). *United States Environmental Protection Agency.*

The many faces of pain. (1996). *Fibromyalgia Network, October.*

The perfume you are wearing may be harmful to your health! (Handout) (1986*). Report by the Committee on science and technology, U.S. House of Representatives.* Report 99-827).

The relationship between prostrate problems and IC is explored. (1996). *ICA Update. The Interstitial Cystitis Association, Fall.*

The right approach to exercise. (1997). *Fibromyalgia Network, July.*

Theohorides, T.C. (1993). Doctor's forum. *The ICA Update. The Interstitial Cystitis Association, Spring.*

Urinary incontinence: Losing control. (Magazine) 1998. *Health and Fitness Magazine, January.*

Urine peptide may contribute to IC. (Internet website) (1999). *Physician Resources. ICA Physician Perspectives, 2.*

Verrilli, G.E., & Mueser, A.M. (1998). *While waiting.* Griffin Trade.

Vliet, E.L. (1995). *Screaming to be heard.* New York: M. Evans and Company.

Webster, D.C. (1993). Sex and Interstitial Cystitis: Explaining the pain and planning self-care. *Urologic Nursing, 13.* 4-11.

Webster, D.C. (1994). Use and effectiveness of physical self-care strategies for Interstitial cystitis. *Nurse Practitioner, October.*

Webster, D.C., & Brennan, T. (1995). Use and effectiveness of sexual self-care strategies for Interstitial Cystitis. *Urologic Nursing, 15.*

What is FMS/CFS? (1996). *Fibromyalgia Network, July.*

Wilson, R.B., Gluck, O.S., Tesser, R.P., Rice, J.C., Meyer, A., & Bridges, A.J. (1999). Antipolymer antibody reactivity in a subset of patients with Fibromyalgia correlates with severity. *The Journal of Rheumatology. 26,* 402-407.

Wilson, R.B. (Handout) (1999). Science summary. Antipolymer antibodies and Fibromylgia syndrome.

Wolfe, S.M. & Hope, R. (1993). *Worst pills best pills II.* (2nd ed.). Washington: Public Citizen's Health Research Group.

Working out in water. (1998). *Harvard Women's Health Watch, May.*

Working with IC. (Internet website) (1999). *ICN Patient Handbook. Interstitial Cystitis Network.*

Ziem, G. (1994). Dr. Grace Ziem's environmental control plan for chemically sensitive patients. Baltimore, MA.

Ziem, G.E. (1992). Multiple chemical sensitivity: Treatment and follow-up with avoidance and control of chemical exposures. *Technology and Industrial Health,* *8,* 73-86.

INDEX

GAYE GRISSOM SANDLER

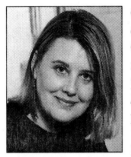

Gaye Grissom Sandler is an author and educator currently living in New Orleans. Gaye has practiced Aston-Patterning movement and muscle re-education for 15 years. She published *Stretch Into a Better Shape,* and in conjunction with the ICA produced a stretching and exercise video in 1993 for IC patients. While living in the Boston area, she facilitated an IC exercise support group for three years at the Newton-Wellesley Hospital. She holds a B.A. in Humanities and completed a two year alternative medicine program at Holistic Life University, one of the first alternative programs in the United States, and became a holistic educator. Gaye has been involved in both traditional and alternative clinics and rehabilitation facilities since 1978.

ANDREW BRENT SANDLER, Ph.D.

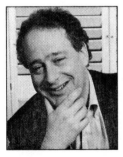

Andrew Brent Sandler has over ten years of clinical and healthcare management experience. He currently holds the position as Administrator of Maison Hospitalière, a nursing home in New Orleans. He has also served in Massachusetts as an Assisted Living Executive Director and as an Alzheimer Program Director. He holds a Ph.D. in Special Education from the University of New Orleans, a Master of Health Administration from Tulane University, an M.A. in Clinical Psychology from Fairleigh Dickinson University, and a B.A. in Psychology from DePauw University. As well as contributing to this book, Andrew presented a Spouse and Family Workshop at the Interstitial Cystitis Association 7th National Meeting in 1993.

TO THE MEMORY OF PRISCILLA NICHOLS